汉英对照《金匮要略》

Chinese-English Textbook
Synopsis of Prescriptions of the Golden Chamber

主　编　阮继源　张光霁
副主编　叶新苗　张　勤　傅　宏
编　委　王　健　金国梁

Chief Editors　Ruan Jiyuan, Zhang Guangji
Assistant Editors　Ye Xinmiao, Zhang Qin, Fu Hong
Compilers　Wang Jian, Jin Guoliang

上海科学技术出版社

图书在版编目（CIP）数据

汉英对照《金匮要略》／阮继源，张光霁主编．—上海：上海科学技术出版社，2003.9
ISBN 7 – 5323 – 7032 – 1

Ⅰ.汉…　Ⅱ.①阮…②张…　Ⅲ.金匮要略方论－汉、英　Ⅳ.R222.3

中国版本图书馆 CIP 数据核字（2003）第031210号

上海科学技术出版社出版发行
（上海瑞金二路 450 号 邮政编码 200020）
常熟市兴达印刷有限公司印刷　新华书店上海发行所经销
2003 年 9 月第 1 版　2003 年 9 月第 1 次印刷
开本 787×1092　1/16　印张 12　字数 257 000
印数 1—3 500　定价：25.00 元

内 容 提 要

　　《金匮要略》是我国现存最早的一部诊治杂病的专书,共有二十五篇,论述了 40 多种疾病,涉及方剂 262 首,是学习中医学必读的一部古典医籍。本书在完全尊重《金匮要略》原文意义的基础上,运用通俗易懂的语言,采用汉英对照的方式,将《金匮要略》全文逐一译成英文,可供中医药院校师生和海外中医药学习者学习《金匮要略》时作为教材使用,亦可供相关学科人员在研究、教学《金匮要略》时作为参考读物。

Abstract

JIN KUI YAO LUE or *Synopsis of Prescriptions of the Golden Chamber* (*SPGC*), As the first clinical medicine classic in China, it attaches much importance to diagnosing miscellaneous disease duo to internal injury. This Classic is divided into 25 chapters and pointing out diagnostic essentials on 40 kinds of diseases according to types of disease, and the classic also deals with 262 prescriptions.

This Chinese-English book is an essential Classic of TCM to read for students. The authors and editors take in the exact definition of the original book, and try to being intelligible, correct and fluent in the English one.

This book can be used by both Foreign and Chinese teachers and students as textbook in all College of Traditional Chinese Medicine, as well as being medical practitioners and scholars in the field as reference books.

何　　序

中医药学是中华民族的宝贵遗产,是一个伟大的宝库。这个伟大的宝库是在特定的历史条件下产生的东方传统医学,它源远流长,内容浩瀚,博大精深,为全世界人民所瞩目。

中医学理论体系初步形成的标志,是先秦秦汉时期所出现的《黄帝内经》、《难经》、《伤寒杂病论》和《神农本草经》等四部医学经典著作。

《黄帝内经》、《难经》奠定了中医学理论体系的基础,《神农本草经》为中医学理论体系提供了较为系统的药物学知识,而作为我国第一部临床医学专著的《伤寒杂病论》以六经辨证和脏腑辨证等方法,对外感疾患和内伤杂病进行了辨证施治,确立了中医临床治疗的辨证论治体系和理、法、方、药等运用原则,为后世临床医学的发展奠定了基础。《伤寒杂病论》经晋代王叔和整理成后世的《伤寒论》和《金匮要略》。

《金匮要略》着重探讨内伤杂病的诊治问题,书中以病分篇,论述了 40 多种疾病的病理特点,分析病变机制,指明诊断要点,全书贯穿着内伤杂病的脏腑辨证方法,并涉及方剂 262 首。其方剂源于临床实践,组方严谨科学,疗效确切,至今仍为国内外临床医师所广泛应用。另外,《金匮要略》发展了《内经》的病因学说,提出"客气邪风,中人多死,千般疢难,不越三条……"初步奠定了中医病因学说的大框架,给后世病因病机学的发展以深刻影响。

近二十年来,随着我国的改革开放,东西文化深层次交流不断深入,作为传统文化灿烂明珠的中医学,作为中国的特色文化要走向世界,为世界人民的健康作出贡献已是迫在眉睫。近年来,《内经》、《伤寒论》等经典医著相继被译成英文等多国文字,走向世界,唯《金匮要略》未见有英译本。1986 年日本东洋学术出版社曾将我的《〈金匮要略〉解说》,翻译成日本文,在日本出版。作为日本学者学习《金匮要略》的教材和参考书,给日本汉方医学界带来很大方便。对于通用英文的域外学习中医学的人们,我想也一定希望能得到《金匮要略》英译本,使得对中国《金匮要略》这一经典古籍内容有进一步、更全面的了解。

阮继源、张光霁两位副教授,在教学、临床及其他专职事务繁重之余,以发扬中医学术、让中医走向世界为己任,策划翻译了《金匮要略》。该书历时之久,用功之深,用心之精,又得翻译名家之指点,实为目下所见英译本著作之佼佼者。须知,要发展中医、弘扬中医,让中医走向世界,不是一句空话,不仅要有所思,而且要有所作为。不积跬步,无以至千里。有志者当如阮继源、张光霁等同志,积极探索,有所创见,为中医学术作出贡献。

何　任

2002 年 11 月 6 日于浙江中医学院

Forword by Heren

Traditional Chinese Medicine (TCM) is a treasure house of Chinese culture heritage. Originated from oriental traditional medicine under special historical situation, it has been increasingly appreciated by the broad masses of the peoples in all parts of the world owing to its long and venerable history, its giant contents and its vast and intensive scope of knowledge.

The four medical classics, *Huangdi's Canon of Medicine*, *Canon on Medical Problems*, *Treatise on Febrile and Miscellaneous Disease*, and *Shen Nong's Canon of Materia Medica*, which all came out around the Qin and Han Dynasty (about 221—206 B.C.) are the milestones marking the initial establishment of the theoretical system of TCM.

On the basis of *Huangdi's Canon of Medicine* and *Canon on Medical Problems*, the theoretical system of Chinese Medicine is provided with systematical knowledge about material medica in *Shen Nong's Canon of Materia Medica*. As the first clinical medical classic in China, *Treatise on Febrile and Miscellaneous Disease* describes various treatments that are made according to diagnosis about exogenous disease and miscellaneous disease due to internal injury, hence a series of principles of applying and so on, and lays a foundation of developing follow-up clinical medicine by means of identifying the symptoms with the names of six channels of Zang and Fu and their interrelation. *Treatise on Febrile and Miscellaneous Disease* was later re-edited by Wang Shuhe in Jin Dynasty into *Treatise on Febrile Disease* and *Synopsis of Prescriptions of Golden Chamber* (*SPGC*).

Synopsis of Prescriptions of the Golden Chamber attaches much importance to diagnosing miscellaneous disease due to internal injury. This Classic is divided into several chapters according to types of diseases, discussing characteristics of pathologic change, and pointing out diagnostic essentials on 40 kinds of diseases around. And the classic also deals with 262 prescriptions and the methods of differentiating diseases according to pathological charges of Zang and Fu and their interrelation. These prescriptions derived from clinical practice. Having been wildly used by clinicians at home and abroad, for they have rigorous scientific approaches and positive curative effects. In addition, The classic *Synopsis of Prescriptions of the Golden Chamber* has developed the etiology theory of *Huangdi's Canon of Medicine*, is almost always due to the three causes that people perish from various diseases, which described in *SPGC*: "When noxious Qi and evil winds attack, death ensues. Even though there are hundreds of thousands of diseases, the causes are three..."laid a preliminary foundation of TCM etiology theory and influenced the later development of etiology and pathogenesis theory.

In the recent 20 years, with the reform and opening to the outside world and further contact between east and west, it's extremely urgent for out TCM, as a shining pearl of the Chinese culture to contribute to the people's health in the world. Lately, many classics of TCM have been translated into English and other languages and disseminated abroad except for English version of *Synopsis of prescriptions of the Golden Chamber*.

In 1986, Toyo academic Press in Japan once translated my *Explanatory Notes to Synopsis of Prescriptions of the Golden Chamber*, as a reference book of learning it into Japanese and published it in Japan, which has benefited the circle of TCM a lot in Japan. In my opinion with an English version of this classic, people, who know English and are eager to learn about some Chinese medicine, will get a further and through understanding of it.

Assistant professor Ruan Jiyuan and Zhang Guangji, took it as his own duty to disseminate TCM throughout the world and schemed for English version of the classic in sprite of his heavy commitment in teaching and clinical work. The amount of the work on this English translation is truly admirable, for Mr. Ruan and Mr. Zhang have taken great pains to accomplish it, spending so much time and energy and trying to obtain guidance and instructions from eminent translators. And this English version is better than other similar one I think, but we must know it should not be a fantasy at all that we should develop TCM and spread it forwards the whole world. Instead, we should not only think about a lot of things, but also attempt some, and accomplish some. "Many a little makes a mickle." People, with lofty ideals of developing TCM, should learn from Mr. Ruan and Mr. Zhang, researching actively, forming some original ideas and making positive achievements for TCM.

Heren

Zhejiang College of Traditional Chinese Medicine

Nov. 6, 2002

前　言

　　《金匮要略》是东汉末年著名医学家张仲景撰写的,是《伤寒杂病论》探讨内伤杂病诊治的部分。《伤寒杂病论》是张仲景在《内经》、《难经》的基础上,进一步总结前人的医学成就,并结合自己的临证经验,写成的我国第一部临床医学专著。它以六经辨证和脏腑辨证等方法,对外感疾患和内伤杂病进行辨证论治,从而确立了中医临床治疗的辨证论治体系和理、法、方、药等运用原则,为后世临床医学的进一步丰富和发展,打下了良好的基础。

　　《伤寒杂病论》经晋代医学家王叔和编纂整理成《伤寒论》和《金匮要略》两书。

　　《金匮要略》着重探讨内伤杂病的诊治问题,书中以病分篇,论述了40多种疾病的病证特点,分析它们的病变机制,指明了诊断要点,全书贯穿着内伤杂病的脏腑辨证方法,并涉及方剂262首。此外,《金匮要略》还发展了《内经》病因学说,提出"千般疢难,不越三条:一者经络受邪入脏腑,为内所因也;二者四肢九窍,血脉相传,壅塞不通,为外皮肤所中也;三者房室金刃虫兽所伤。以此详之,病由都尽。"给后世包括《三因极一病证方论》的病因病机学的发展以深刻影响。

　　《伤寒杂病论》奠定了中医学辨证论治理论体系的基础,是中医学的经典著作之一,作为其重要组成部分的《金匮要略》,其地位不用赘述。

　　正是由于《金匮要略》对中医临床的重要意义,历代医学家不仅重视,而且往往倾注大量精力予以研究,直至当代,仍有许多医学家在孜孜不倦地研究《金匮要略》,涌现出了许多的金匮专家,产生了很多的成果,譬如以被日本人称为"当今金匮第一人"——何任老教授为首的课题组,他们的研究成果《〈金匮要略〉校法》获国家卫生部科技进步二等奖。在何老的带领下,浙江中医学院也形成了以《金匮要略》研究为特色的中医临床基础学科,学科先后被评为浙江省重点学科和国家中医药管理局重点学科建设单位。

　　查诸文献,《内经》、《伤寒论》等经典医著都已有英译本,唯《金匮要略》未见有英译本。我们为浙江中医学院的一员,又习岐黄之道,自感肩上责任重大,有义务让《金匮要略》英译本问世,为中医现代化、为中医文化走向世界尽绵薄之力,所以我们策划翻译了这本《金匮要略》英译本。为求对原文的准确理解,我们选用了李克光主编的《〈金匮要略〉译释》(上海科学技术出版社,1993年4月,第一版)为中文底本,历时5年,终于译成初稿。本书承蒙原浙江大学外语系主任庄根源教授的厚爱,为之审校;承蒙第一批国家级名老中医、著名金匮专家何任教授的厚爱,为之作序;承蒙浙江省书法家协会会员石云先生不吝赐墨,题写书名,在此,一并对所有关心、支持本书翻译、出版的同志同致谢忱。

但水平有限，又是第一次全书将中文翻译成英文，难免存在着许多不足之处，望读者予以批评，以利于我们在再版时予以更正与完善。

阮继源　张光霁

2002 年 11 月 6 日于浙江中医学院

Preface

Synopsis of prescriptions of the Golden Chamber, composed by Zhang Zhongjing, on eminent medical scientist in the late Donghan Dynasty, is a section of *Treatise on Febrile and Miscellaneous Disease*, a section focused on discussing diagnosis of miscellaneous diseases due to internal injury.

As the first clinical medical classic in China, *Treatise on Febrile and miscellaneous Disease* describes various treatments that are made according to diagnosis about exogenous disease and miscellaneous disease due to internal injury, hence a series of principles of applying and so on, and lays a foundation of developing follow-up clinical medicine by means of identifying the symptoms with the names of six channels of Zang and Fu and their interrelation. *Treatise on Febrile and Miscellaneous Disease* was later re-edited by Wang Shuhe in Jin Dynasty into *Treatise on Febrile Disease* and *Synopsis of Prescriptions of Golden Chamber*.

Synopsis of prescriptions of the Golden Chamber attaches much importance to diagnosing miscellaneous diseases due to internal injury. This Classic is divided into several chapters according to types of diseases, discussing characteristics of pathology, analysizing mechanism of pathologic change, and pointing out diagnostic essentials on 40 kinds of diseases around. And the classic also deals with 262 prescriptions and the methods of differentiating diseases according to pathological changes of Zang and Fu and their interrelation. In addition, the classic has developed the etiology theory of *Huangdi's Canon of Medicine*, claiming that "it is almost always due to the three causes that people perish from various diseases though there are hundreds of thousands of diseases: ① internal evils spreading along the meridians to the Zang and Fu. ② external evils breaking through the surface of the skin and invading the interior (eventually the evils cause blockage of the blood and Qi in the four limbs and the nine cavities). ③ sexual abuse, knife wounds, and animal or insect bits." That laid a preliminary foundation of TCM etiology theory and influence the later development of etiology and pathogenesis theory, such as that of *Treatise on Three Categories of Pathogenic Factors and Symptoms*. It is owing to the great clinical significance of *Synopsis of Prescriptions of the Golden Chamber* (*SPGC*) that physicians of various historical periods have attached so much importance to it, even up to now, spending great energy in doing researches in it, and a great many experts yielding with admirable achievements in this field during the cause such as Heren, who is known by Japanese as "the first person" – most eminent figure in the study of *SPGC* at present. His research achievement – *Proofread of Synopsis of prescription of the Golden Chamber*, was awarded with a silver medal of the scientific progress Prize melted out by Ministry of Health P. R. China.

Under his leadership, Zhejiang College of TCM has established a primary course of TCM Clinics characterized by the study of *SPGC*, which was appointed as a key course of Zhejiang province and, also, one of the key courses to be enhanced by the State Administration of TCM P. R. China.

Many classics of TCM have been translated into English except *SPGC*. Being a member of Zhejiang College of TCM, we find it our duty to translate the classic into English, so as to do our bit for the cause of modernizing TCM and disseminating it through out the world. So we schemed for the translation of *SPGC* into English. In order to take in the exact definition of the original, we choose *Explanatory Notes of SPGC* as text proper for our translation (chiefly compiled by Li Keguang, Shanghai Scientific and Technical Publishers, Apr. 1993, first published), It took us five years to finish the first draft.

We would like to express special appreciation to Professor Zhuang Genyuan, pre-dean of foreign language Institute in Zhejiang University, for this providing a through proofing and review of the book to professor Heren, a-first-rate State Veteran TCM Doctor, for his writing the forward, to Mr. Siyun, a member of Calligrapher association of Zhejiang Province, for his inscribing the book's name and to others for their support and help. It's difficult to achieve the desired results because of the lack of experience, the limited knowledge and the difficulty involved in this initial effort to translate the whole book. We, therefore, appreciate sincerely the valuable suggestions and advise from scholars at home and abroad so as to make further improvement and revision.

Ruan Jiyuan, Zhang Guangji

Zhejiang College of Traditional Chinese Medicine

Nov. 6,2002

目　录

CONTENT

脏腑经络先后病脉证第一

I.

On Pulse Syndrome Complex and Transmission of the Disease of Viscera, Bowels, Channels and Collaterals

第一节　问曰:上工治未病,何也? 师曰:夫治未病者,见肝之病,知肝传脾,当先实脾。四季脾旺不受邪,即勿补之。中工不晓相传,见肝之病,不解实脾,惟治肝也。夫肝之病,补用酸,助用焦苦,益用甘味之药调之。酸入肝,焦苦入心,甘入脾,脾能伤肾,肾气微弱,则水不行;水不行,则心火气盛,则伤肺;肺被伤,则金气不行;金气不行,则肝气盛,则肝自愈。此治肝补脾之要妙也。肝虚则用此法,实则不在用之。经曰"虚虚实实,补不足,损有余。"是其义也。余藏准此。

1. The disciples asked: "Why does a superior physician treat disease before its onset?" The master replied: "Because to treat a disease before its onset means that liver disease eventually transmits to the spleen; therefore he takes care to maintain the strength of the spleen. However, in the last month of a season when the spleen is vigorous and will not contract any ailment, it is unnecessary to supplement the spleen. A mediocre physician, not understanding transmission, treats only the liver without strengthening the spleen."

In treating liver disorders sour herbs supplement the liver; charred, bitter herbs assist the heart; and sweet herbs harmonize the spleen. The rule is based on the principle that sour drugs enter the liver; charred, bitter drugs, the heart; and sweet drugs, the spleen. A strengthened spleen overworks and thus overloads the kidney; the latter then weakens and no longer releases water. Hindered water flow causes heart fire to thrive and injure the lung. Once the lung is injured, plumonary Qi will not act. The deactivation of metal Qi leads to exuberance of liver Qi and spontaneous recovery of the liver. This is an effective way to treat the liver and supplement the spleen. This method, however, is only applicable to the deficiency syndrome of the liver, but not to the excess syndrome of the liver. The Canon says: "Disease conditions vary – some are of deficiency while others are of excess. Correct treatment is to supplement insufficiency and purge excess." This example illustrates a medical principle applicable to other visceral disorders.

第二节　夫人禀五常,因风气而生长。风气虽能生万物,亦能害万物,如水能浮舟,亦能覆舟。若五脏元真通畅,人即安和。客气邪风,中人多死。千般疢难,不越三条:一者,经络受邪入脏腑为内所因也;二者,四肢九窍,血脉相传,壅塞不通,为外皮肤所中也;三者,房室、金刃、虫兽所伤,以此详之,病由都尽。若人能养慎,不令邪风干忤经络;适中经络,未流传脏腑,即医治之;四肢才觉重滞,即导引吐纳、针灸、膏摩,勿令九窍闭塞;更能无犯王法、禽兽疢伤;房室勿令竭乏,服食节其冷热苦酸辛甘,不遗形体有衰,病则无由入其腠理。腠者,是三焦通会元真之处,为血气所注;理者,是皮肤脏腑之文理也。

2. Climate greatly influences the five organs (viscera) with which the human being is endowed. Nature nourishes and destroys all creatures just as water both floats and overturn a ship. When the primordial Qi of the five viscera circulates smoothly, the body remains healthy and well; but when noxious Qi and evil winds attack, death ensues. Even though there are hundreds of thousands of diseases, the causes are three: ① internal evils spreading along the meridians to the viscera. ② external evils breaking through the surface of the skin and invading the interior (eventually the evils cause blockage of the blood and Qi in the four limbs and the nine cavities). ③ sexual abuse, knife wounds, and animal or insect bites. All diseases fall into one of these categories. Disease can not invade the cou li (interstices) if one lives circumspectly.

Disease should be treated immediately before the meridians are involved and the viscera harmed. The immediate practice of Qi guidance exercises, tuina, acupuncture and moxibustion, or unguent massage prevents obstruction of the nine cavities and thus relieve feelings of heaviness and torpidity. One should behave so as not to violate the law or to incur injuries from animals. One should not exhaust oneself in sexual indulgence, and one should always wear proper clothing, so as not to become too hot or too cold. Finally, one should cultivate proper eating habits and balance the eating of sweet, bitter, and sour foods.

第三节　问曰:病人有气色见于面部,愿闻其说。师曰:鼻头色青,腹中痛,苦冷者死;鼻头色微黑者,有水气;色黄者,胸上有寒;色白者,亡血也,设微赤非时者,死。其目正圆者痉("痉"原作"痓"),不治。又色青为痛,色黑为劳。色赤为风,色黄者便难,色鲜明者有留饮。

3. The disciples asked: "Would you instruct us on the colors of Qi that exhibit themselves in the facial complexion?"

The master replied: "When the tip of the nose looks green, it signifies abdominal aching. If the patient also feels chilly and aches painfully, he is in critical condition. When the tip of the nose appears slightly black, it denotes the presence of moisture. Yellow indicates chills (water stagnancy) in the chest and a white nose signals blood loss. A patient with a slightly red facial complexion in a season incongruent with the color – red corresponds to hot weather or the summer – is in critical condition. Fixed and motionless eyes occur with critical spasms. A green facial complexion accompanies aching; a black facial complexion, consumptive disease; and a red complexion, wind disease. A yellow complexion denotes constipation, and a bright, lustrous complexion accompanies water stagnancy (edema)."

第四节　师曰:病人语声寂然喜惊呼者,骨节间病;语声喑喑然不彻者,心膈间病;语声啾啾然细而长者,头中病。

4. The master said: "A quiet person who occasionally cries out has joint disease whereas a person with a low, unclear voice has a problem between the diaphragm and the heart. A thin, draw-out voice indicates brain disease."

第五节　师曰:息摇肩者心中坚;息引胸中上气者,咳;息张口短气者,肺痿唾沫。

5. The master said: "A patient with difficult breathing causing drawn shoulders has a firm chest obstruction. Adverse welling up of Qi causes coughing. If the patient gasps for air with a wide open mouth when he breathes and if he expectorates frothy sputum, pulmonary atrophy has set in."

第六节　师曰:吸而微数,其病在中焦实也,当下之即愈;虚者不治。在上焦者,其吸促,在下焦者,其吸远;此皆难治。呼吸动摇振振者,不治。

6. The master said: "Slightly rapid respiration means the problem is firm evil located in the middle warmer; purgation heals the condition. In a patient with a weak conformation, the condition is harder to cure. If the evil is located in the upper warmer, breathing will be short and shallow. If the evil is located in the lower warmer, the breathing will be deep and slow. Both conditions resist therapy. If the patient's body shakes while breathing, the condition is also difficult to treat."

第七节　师曰:寸口脉动者,因其旺时而动,假令肝旺色青,四时各随其色。肝色青而反色白,非其时色脉,皆当病。

7. The master said: "Pulse at cunkou will follow the changes in Vital Energy of a certain Viscus in different seasons. Vital Energy of the Viscera will appear as different colors when they are strong in certain seasons. For example, blue-purple (cyanosis) signifies strong Vital Energy in the Liver. Under normal conditions, the four seasons will give birth to their respective colors. When blue-purple (cyanosis) of the Liver Vital Energy does not appear as it should, but white (pallor) color appears, it is an indication of disease. In all cases when unseasonal colors or pulses appear,

they can be diagnosed as symptoms and signs of diseases."

第八节 问曰:有未至而至,有至而不至,有至而不去,有至而太过,何谓也? 师曰:冬至之后,甲子夜半少阳起,少阳之时阳始生,天得温和。以未得甲子,天因温和,此为未至而至也;以得甲子,而天未温和,此为至而不至也;以得甲子,而天未温和,为至而不至也;以得甲子,而天大寒不解,此为至而不去也;以得甲子,而天温如盛夏五六月时,此为至而太过也。

8. The disciples asked: "Tell us why the seasons arrive at various times; sometimes a season arrives before the calendar date, sometimes after; or sometimes the calendar date arrives but the preceding season remains; or sometimes the season arrives before its time."

The master replied: "Exactly at midnight on the winter solstice, the lesser yang period begins, that is, the yang phase is setting in; thence the weather gradually warms. If the weather becomes warm before the winter solstice, it is the first condition. If the winter solstice arrives but the weather has not turned warm, it is the second condition. If the winter solstice arrives but the weather remaines extremely chilly and there is no sign of warm weather, it is the third condition. If the calendrical winter solstice arrives, but it is as hot as midsummer, it is the fourth condition."

第九节 师曰:病人脉浮者在前,其病在表;浮者在后,其病在里,腰痛背强不能行,必短气而极也。

9. The master said: "A floating pulse on the cun site before the guan reflects a surface problem. A floating pulse on the chi site behind the guan signifies an internal disease whereby the patient will have low back pain, a stiff back, lameness, and the development of critical gasping."

第十节 问曰:经云"厥阳独行",何谓也? 师曰:此为有阳无阴,故称厥阳。

10. The disciples asked: "What is the *meaning* of the exuberant Yang Prevails and moves about alone as it says in *Huangdi's canon of medicine*?"

The master said: "This is because when the exuberant Yang prevails, there Will be no Yin. and Yang moves alone So it is called Jue Yang."

第十一节 问曰:寸脉沉大而滑,沉则为实,滑则为气,实气相搏,血气入脏即死,入腑即愈,此为卒厥,何谓也? 师曰:唇口青,身冷,为入脏即死;如身和,汗自出,为入腑即愈。

11. The disciples said: "When the pulse on the cun site is submerged, big, and slippery wherein 'submerged' signifies blood firmness and 'slippery' Qi firmness, the firmness evils are in-

teracting forcing blood and Qi into the viscera. This condition results in death or recovery depending on the viscera involved. Why is the condition called 'sudden faint?'"

The master answered: "A blue-tinged mouth and general chills indicate that evils are in the solid viscera (zang) and the patient will die. On the other hand, a balanced body with spontaneous perspiration indicates that the evils are in the hollow viscera (fu) and the patient will recover."

第十二节　问曰:脉脱入脏即死,入腑即愈,何谓也? 师曰:非为一病,百病皆然。譬如浸淫疮,从口起流向四肢者可治,从四肢流来入口者不可治,病在外者可治,入里者即死。

12. The disciples asked: "If the patient occasionally shows a sudden absence of pulse, he will die, the evil has entered the solid viscera. If the evil has entered the hollow viscera, he will survive and recover. Why so?"

The master said: "This rule applies not only to evil illness but to all diseases. Take for example, spreading skin sores. If the disease starts at the mouth and spreads to the four limbs (from the interior toward the exterior), the condition is curable. But if the disease starts in the limbs and moves toward the mouth, the condition is incurable. Exterior diseases are curable, whereas diseases that have penetrated the interior are lethal."

第十三节　问曰:阳病十八,何谓也? 师曰:头痛、项、腰、脊、臂、脚掣痛。阴病十八,何谓也? 师曰:咳、上气、喘、哕、咽、肠鸣、胀满、心痛、拘急。五脏病各有十八,合为九十病,人又有六微,微有十八病,合为一百八病。五劳、七伤、六极、妇人三十六病,不在其中。清邪居上,浊邪居下,大邪中表,小邪中里,槃饪之邪,从口入者,宿食也。五邪中人,各有法度,风中于前,寒中于暮,湿伤于下,雾伤于上,风令脉浮,寒令脉急,雾伤皮腠,湿流关节,食伤脾胃,极寒伤经,极热伤络。

13. The disciples asked: "Why are there eighteen yang diseases and eighteen yin diseases?"

The master said: "Symptoms such as headache or dragging pains of the neck, waist, spine, arms, and feet indicate yang diseases (six yang symptoms) because they are surface and 'meridional' coughing, asthma due to flushing of Qi, retching pharyngeal obstruction, borborygmus with abdominal distention, and cardialgia with spasms, indicate yin diseases (six yin symptoms) because the symptoms are internal and visceral. The yang diseases are differentiated into lesser yang, sunlight yang, and greater yang; three (types) times six (symptoms) is eighteen. Thus there are eighteen yang diseases. On the other hand, yin diseases are differentiated into lesser yin, greater yin, and absolute yin; three (types) times six (symptoms) is eighteen. Thus there are also eighteen yin diseases. Since there are five solid organs in the body and each of them is susceptible to eighteen diseases, the number of yin and yang diseases each totals ninety. Six mild diseases derive from the mild evils. They invade the six hollow viscera and come in three types. Thus there are another eighteen diseases; therefore there are a total of one hundred and eight diseases of the hollow viscera. The above diseases do not include ailments caused by the five fatigues, the seven emotions, the six culminations, and the thirty-six problems of women.

"Clear evils attack above the waist, turbid evils below; the severe evils occur superficially; the mild evils, internally; and the evils from the poorly prepared food eaten cause indigestion overnight. The five evils – wind, cold, moisture, fog, and food – afflict the body in definite ways. Wind evils strike in the forenoon; cold evils at dusk. Moisture evils affect the lower torso, while fog evils invade the upper torso. Wind evils cause a floating pulse and chill evils, a quick pulse. Fog evils injure the skin and muscles. Moisture evils immobilize the joints. Inappropriate food injures the stomach and spleen; extreme chill, the longitudinal or internal meridians (Jing); and extreme heat, the transverse or surface meridians (luo)."

第十四节　问曰:病有急当救里救表者,何谓也? 师曰:病,医下之,续得下利清谷不止,身体疼痛者,急当救里;后身体疼痛,清便自调者,急当救表也。

14. The disciples asked: "What is the priority of treatment in the simultaneous presence of surface and internal symptoms?"

The master said: "If after a purgative treatment the patient has incessant lientery and generalized aching, the internal symptom of lientery must be treated first. If after treatment the lientery has stopped but the generalized aching remains unrelieved, the aching, which is a surface symptom, must then be treated at once."

第十五节　夫病痼疾加以卒病,当先治其卒病,后乃治其痼疾也。

15. The master admonished: "When a patient who has been suffering from a chronic disease suddenly incurs an acute disease, it is mandatory to begin treating the acute disease before addressing the chronic condition."

第十六节　师曰:五脏病各有得者愈,五脏病各有所恶,各随其所不喜者为病。病者素不应食,而反暴思之,必发热也。

16. The master said: "Each visceral disease has its own specific environment and conditions appropriate for recovery. Contrarily, each visceral disease also has its own uncongenial environment and inappropriate conditions for contracting the disease. For instance, a patient who suddenly craves some food which he previously did not even like may develop a fever after eating that food."

第十七节　夫诸病在脏,欲攻之,当随其所得而攻之,如渴者,与猪苓汤。余皆仿此。

猪苓汤方:猪苓(去皮)、茯苓、阿胶、滑石、泽泻各一两。

上五味,以水四升,先煮四味,取二升,去滓,内胶烊消,温服七合,日三服。

17. While the disease is affecting the Viscera, attacking or purgative therapy is appropriate only when corresponding symptoms and signs are observed. For instance, if the patient is thirsty for water, Decoction of Polyporus Umbellatus (Zhu ling-tang) can be administered. Similar treatment can be applied for all other cases.

1 liang decorticated polyporus.　　　　1 liang talc

1 liang hoelen　　　　　　　　　　　1 liang alisma

1 liang gelatin

Decoct all ingredients except gelatin in 4 sheng of water until 2 sheng remains. Discard the dregs and dissolve the gelatin in the decoction. Seven-tenths sheng is warmed and taken three times daily.

痉湿暍病脉证治第二

II.

On Pulse Syndrome Complex and Treatment of Convulsion, Moisture Disease(Rheumatism), and Heatstroke

第一节　太阳病,发热无汗,反恶寒者,名曰刚痉。

1. One type of Initial Yang syndrome with symptoms and signs of fever, no perspiration , but aversion to cold is termed GangJing(strong convulsions).

第二节　太阳病,发热汗出,而不恶寒,名曰柔痉。

2. Another type of Initial Yang syndrome with symptoms and signs of fever and perspiration, but with no aversion to cold, is termed RouJing(weak convulsions).

第三节　太阳病,发热,脉沉而细者,名曰痉,为难治。

3. Initial Yang syndrome with fever, a submerged and thin pulse, and muscle spasms is termed Jing disease(convulsions), and is difficult to cure.

第四节　太阳病,发汗太多,因致痉。

4. Initial Yang syndrome: Profuse perspiration will cause a Jing disease.

第五节　夫风病,下之则痉,复发汗,必拘急。

5. A wind disease improperly treated by purgation produces convulsions. The inducement of perspiring also results in spasms in the arms and legs.

第六节　疮家虽身疼痛,不可发汗,汗出则痓。

6. Thus a patient suffering from sores, despite his generalized aching, should not be sweated because it will cause convulsions.

第七节　病者身热足寒,颈项强急,恶寒,时头热,面赤,目赤,独头动摇,卒口噤,背反张者,痓病也。若发其汗者,寒湿相得,其表益虚,即恶寒甚。发其汗已,其脉如蛇。

7. A convulsive (Jing) disease manifests the symptoms of generalized fever, cold feet, stiff neck, chillphobia, occasional head fever, facial and ocular hyperemia, involuntary shaking of the head, lockjaw, and tetany. If the patient is sweated, the chill and moisture evils will interact causing further weakening of the surface and more severe chillphobia. After sweating, the patient's pulse becomes like a writhing snake.

第八节　暴腹胀大者,为欲解,脉如故,反伏弦者,痓。

8. When a patient suffering from a Jing disease suddenly feels abdominal distention, it is a sign of recovery. If the pulse remains the same but if the pulse becomes hidden and chordal, convulsive disease has set in.

第九节　夫痓脉,按之紧如弦,直上下行。

9. The pulse in convulsive diseases feels as tense as a chord and is palpable all the way from the upper (cun) to the lower (chi) site.

第十节　痓病有灸疮,难治。

10. Convulsions in a patient with sores are difficult to arrest.

第十一节　太阳病,其证备,身体强,几几然,脉反沉迟,此为痓,栝蒌桂枝汤主之。
栝蒌桂枝汤方:栝蒌根二两,桂枝三两(去皮),芍药三两,甘草二两(炙),生姜三两(切),大枣十二枚(擘)。上六味,以水九升,煮取三升,分温三服,取微汗。汗不出,食顷,啜热粥发之。

11. The conformation of a convulsive disease includes the complete symptoms of Initial Yang syndrome together with a rigid body, stiff neck and back, and a submerged and slow pulse. It should be treated primarily with Gua-lou-gui-zhi-tang (Trichosanthes and Cinnamon Combination).

3 liang trichosanthes root	2 liang baked licorice
3 liang decorticated cinnamon	3 liang cut fresh ginger
3 liang peony	12 pcs. smashed jujube fruits

Boil the ingredients in 9 sheng of water until 3 sheng remains. Divide the solution into three portions. A warmed portion should produce mild perspiring. If no perspiring occurs, sip hot rice congee after drinking the herb decoction.

第十二节　太阳病,无汗而小便反少,气上冲胸,口噤不得语,欲作刚痉,葛根汤主之。

葛根汤方:葛根四两,麻黄三两(去节),桂枝二两(去皮),芍药二两,甘草二两(炙),生姜三两(切),大枣十二枚(擘)。上七味,㕮咀,以水一斗(一作"七升"),先煮麻黄、葛根,减二升,去沫。内诸药,煮取三升,去滓,温服一升,覆取微似汗,不须啜粥,余如桂枝汤将息及禁忌。

12. Initial Yang syndrome with anhidrosis, oliguria, flushing of Qi toward the chest, lockjaw, and a tendency to have strong convulsions should be treated with Ge-gen-tang (Pueraria Combination).

4 liang pueraria	2 liang baked licorice
3 liang denoded mahuang	3 liang cut fresh ginger
2 liang decorticated cinnamon	12 pcs. smashed jujube fruit
2 liang peony	

After the ingredients are cut up, boil the mahuang and pueraria with 10 sheng of water until the volume has been reduced by 2 sheng. Then skim off the foam, add the other herbs, and boil until 3 sheng remains. Drain the solution and discard the dregs. One sheng warmed of the decoction constitutes a dose. The patient should be wrapped in a quilt to make him perspire (without sipping rice congee). The same instructions for administration and contraindications apply as for Gui-zhi-tang (Cinnamon Combination).

3 liang decorticated cinnamon	3 liang fresh ginger
3 liang peony	12 jujube fruits
2 liang baked licorice	

Shred the ingredients and decoct in 7 sheng of water on a mild fire until 3 sheng remains. Discard the dregs. One sheng of the decoction taken at the appropriate temperature followed by sipping 1 sheng of thin rice congee a short while later will augment the drug's effect. The patient should be mildly sweated by wrapping him in a quilt for about three hours. Heavy sweating should be avoided. If the patient perspires and heals after taking the first portion of decoction, the remaining portions are suspended. If he does not sweat, the remaining portions are taken in the same way as indicated for the first one. The patient should not eat raw or cold food, noodles, wine, or cheese while he is under treatment with this formula.

第十三节　痉为病。胸满,口噤,卧不着席,脚挛急,必龂齿,可与大承气汤。

大承气汤方:大黄四两(酒洗),厚朴半斤(炙去皮),枳实五枚(炙),芒硝三合。上四味,以水一斗,先煮二物,取五升,去滓,内大黄,煮取二升,去滓,内芒硝,更上微火一二沸,分温再服,得下止服。

13. A strong convulsive disease in a patient manifesting thoracic fullness, lockjaw, tetany, spasms of the feet, and involuntary gnashing of teeth may be treated with Da-cheng-qi-tang(Major Rhubarb Combination).

4 liang wine-washed rhubarb	5 pcs. zhi-shi fruits
0.5 jin seared magnolia with outer bark removed	3 ge mirabilitum

Decoct the magnolia and zhi-shi in 10 sheng of water until 5 sheng remains. Remove the sediment and add the rhubarb. Boil again until 2 sheng remains. Discard the dregs, add the mirabilitum, and reboil on a mild fire for a short time. The decoction is divided into two portions, and each portion is taken warmed. If bowel movement occurs, the subsequent dose is suspended.

第十四节　太阳病,关节疼痛而烦,脉沉而细者,此名湿痹。湿痹之候,小便不利,大便反快,但当利其小便。

14. Initial Yang syndrome exhibiting arthralgia, distress, and a submerged and thin pulse is known as moist disease(rheumatism). It should be treated with a diuretic when there is oliguria and diarrhea.

第十五节　湿家之为病,一身尽疼。发热,身色如熏黄也。

15. Patients with moisture disease suffer from generalized aching and fever and exhibit a smoky yellow discoloration of the whole body.

第十六节　湿家,其人但头汗出,背强,欲得被覆向火。若下之早则哕,或胸满,小便不利,舌上如胎者,以丹田有热,胸上有寒,渴欲得饮而不能饮,则口燥烦也。

16. Patients suffering from moisture disease who perspire on the head only, have a stiff back, and wish to be wrapped in a quilt or to sit close to a fire will retch or develop chest fullness, oliguria, and fur-like tongue coating if purgation is conducted prematurely. A fever in the lower torso and chill in the chest causes thirst and a dry mouth. The afflicted have a desire to drink liquids but cannot.

第十七节　湿家下之,额上汗出,微喘,小便利者死;若下利不止者,亦死。

17. In a patient with moisture disease if purgation causes perspiring of the forehead, mild gasping, and polyuria, the patient will die. Also, if incessant diarrhea results, the patient will die.

第十八节　风湿相搏,一身尽疼痛,法当汗出而解,值天阴雨不止,医云此可发汗,汗之病不愈者,何也? 盖发其汗,汗大出者,但风气去,湿气在,是故不愈也。若治风湿者,发其汗,但微微似欲汗出者,风湿俱去也。

18. Interaction between wind and moisture evils causes generalized aching which can be resolved by the sweating method. However, once a physician treated the condition with the sweating method on a rainy day, but the patient did not recover. Why? Because the profuse sweating only eliminated the wind evil while the moisture evil remained; thus the patient was not cured. The correct way of treating wind and moisture evils (rhuematism) is to instigate mild perspiring. In this way both wind and moisture evils will be eliminated.

第十九节　湿家病身疼发热,面黄而喘,头痛鼻塞而烦,其脉大,自能饮食,腹中和无病,病在头中寒湿,故鼻塞,内药鼻中则愈。

19. A patient with moisture disease manifesting generalized aching, fever, a yellowish facial complexion, asthma, headache, stuffy nose, distress, and a big pulse but normal eating and drinking, a harmonious abdominal condition, and cold-dampness disease in the head. The stuffy nose can be cured by placing medication in the patient's nose.

第二十节　湿家身烦疼,可与麻黄加术汤发其汗为宜,慎不可以火攻之。

麻黄加术汤方:麻黄三两(去节),桂枝二两(去皮),甘草一两(炙),杏仁七十个(去皮尖),白术四两。上五味,以水九升,先煮麻黄,减二升,去上沫,内诸药,煮取二升半,去滓,温服八合,覆取微似汗。

20. A patient with moisture disease manifesting generalized vexation and aching may be suitably treated by inducing sweating with Ma-huang-jia-shu-tang (Mahuang and Atractylodes Combination). The doctor should be cautioned against using the fire-attacking method.

3 liang denoded mahuang

2 liang decorticated cinnamon

1 liang baked licorice

70 pcs. apricot seeds with the apex and outer skin removed

4 liang atractylodes

First boil mahuang with 9 sheng of water until the volume has reduced by 2 sheng. Skim the foam off, add the other herbs, and boil until 2 sheng remains. After discarding the dregs, the patient should drink 0.8 sheng of the decoction warm and cover himself with quilts to bring about mild perspiring.

第二十一节　病者一身尽疼,发热,日晡所剧者,名风湿。此病伤于汗出当风,或久伤取冷所致也。可与麻黄杏仁薏苡甘草汤。

麻黄杏仁薏苡甘草汤方:麻黄(去节)半两(汤泡),甘草一两(炙),薏苡仁半两,杏仁十个(去皮尖,炒)。上剉麻豆大,每服四钱匕,水盏半,煮八分,去滓,温服,有微汗,避风。

21. Generalized aching and fever which aggravates in the evening also accompanies rheumatism. It occurs when one who is perspiring is caught in a draft or when one gets cold in the presence of a chronic injury. Treatment calls for Ma-xing-yi-gan-tang (Mahuang and Coix Combination).

0.5 liang denoded and water-soaked mahuang　　　　1 liang baked licorice

10 pcs. fried apricot seeds with the apex and outer skin removed　　0.5 liang coix

Chop up the drugs. Allow four qianbi for each dose. Stew the drugs in one and a half cups of water until eight fen remain. Filter the decoction and serve warm to induce a light perspiration. Keep the patient away from wind.

第二十二节　风湿,脉浮、身重、汗出恶风者,防己黄芪汤主之。

防己黄芪汤方:防己一两,甘草半两(炒),白术七钱半,黄芪一两一分(去芦)。上剉麻豆大,每抄五钱匕,生姜四片,大枣一枚,水盏半,煎八分,去滓,温服,良久再服。喘者加麻黄半两,胃中不和者加芍药三分,气上冲者加桂枝三分,下有陈寒者加细辛三分。服后当如虫行皮中,从腰下如冰,后坐被上,又以一被绕腰以下,温令微汗,差。

22. Fang-ji-huang-qi-tang (Stephania and Astragalus Combination) treats rheumatism with a floating pulse, generalized heaviness, sweating, and anemophobia.

1 liang stephania　　　　　　　　1 liang and 1 fen astragalus (remove the stem remnant)

0.5 liang fried licorice

0.75 liang atractylodes

Chop up the drugs. Five qianbi per dose. Stew in one and a half cups water with four pieces of Rhizoma Zingiberis Recens and one piece of Fructus Ziziphi Jujubae until eight fen remain. Filter the decoction and serve warm. A second dose can be served after along interval. For the patients with asthma, add 0.5 liang of mahuang; for gastric disharmony, 3 fen of peony; for flushing of Qi, 3 fen of cinnamon; and for chronic chills in the lower body, 3 fen of asarum. After drinking the decoction, the patient feels as if worms were crawling in his skin and the area from the waist to the feet becomes as cold as ice. The patient should sit on quilts and be wrapped in another quilt below the waist so that he keeps warm enough to produce mild perspiration, thus promoting recovery.

第二十三节　伤寒,八九日,风湿相搏,身体疼烦,不能自转侧,不呕不渴,脉浮虚而涩者,桂枝附子汤主之;若大便坚,小便自利者。去桂加白术汤主之。

桂枝附子汤方:桂枝四两(去皮),生姜三两(切),附子三枚(炮去皮,破八片),甘草二两(炙),大枣十二枚(擘)。上五味,以水六升煮取二升,去滓,分温三服。

白术附子汤方:白术二两,附子一枚半(炮去皮),甘草一两(炙),生姜一两半(切),大枣六枚(擘)。上五味,以水三升,煮取一升,去滓,分温三服。一服觉身痹,半日许再服,三服都尽,其人如冒状,勿怪,即是术、附并走皮中,逐水气,未得除故耳。

23. A shang han condition that has lasted for eight to nine days with wind and moisture evils interacting-generalized aching and vexation, inability to turn over voluntarily, no vomiting, no thirst, and a floating, empty, and harsh pulse requires the basic treatment of Gui-zhi-fu-zhi-tang (Cinnamon, Aconite, and Ginger Combination).

4 liang decorticated cinnamon　　　　　3 liang cut fresh ginger

2 liang baked licorice　　　　　　　　3 pcs. aconite roots (baked, skinned, and

12 pcs. smashed jujube fruits　　　　　broken it into 8 pieces each)

Decoct the ingredients in 6 sheng of water until 2 sheng remains, discard the dregs, and divide the decoction in three portions. Take each portion warmed.

If the patient has constipation and polyuria, Bai-shu-fu-zhi-tang (Atractylodes and Aconite Combination) is the principal treatment.

2 liang atractylodes　　　　　　　　　1 liang baked licorice

1.5 pcs. aconite roots baked to remove　1.5 liang cut fresh ginger

the outer skin　　　　　　　　　　　6 pcs. smashed jujube fruits

Decoct the ingredients in 3 sheng of water until 1 sheng remains. Discard the dregs and divide the decoction into three portions. It should be taken warmed. The first portion will produce a generalized paralytic sensation. The second and third portions following at intervals of half a day will cause dizziness. Do not be alarmed by this phenomenon. It is due to the atractylodes and aconite acting in the skin and not having completely driven off the water vapor.

第二十四节　风湿相搏,骨节疼烦掣痛,不得屈伸,近之则痛剧,汗出短气,小便不利,恶风,不欲去衣,或身微肿者,甘草附子汤主之。

甘草附子汤方:甘草二两(炙),白术二两,附子二枚(炮去皮),桂枝四两(去皮)。上四味,以水六升煮取三升,去滓。温服一升,日三服,初服得微汗则解,能食,汗出复烦者,服五合。恐一升多者,服六、七合为妙。

24. An interaction between wind and moisture toxins that causes arthralgia, spasmodic pain, inability to flex and stretch, severe pain upon touching, sweating, gasping, oliguria, anemophobia

to the point of disliking to undress even, or mild generalied edema should be treated principally with Gan-cao-fu-zhi-tang(Licorice and Aconite Combination).

2 liang baked licorice

2 liang atractylodes

1 pcs. aconite root baked with the bark removed

4 liang cinnamon with the bark removed

Decoct the four ingredients with 6 sheng of water until 3 sheng remains. Drain and discard the dregs. One sheng is taken three times daily. If mild perspiring occurs after the first dose, the problem will resolve and the patient will have an appetite, If vexation follows perspiring, 5 ge more is taken. One sheng may be too much; then 6 – 7 ge is all right.

第二十五节　太阳中暍,发热恶寒,身重而疼痛,其脉弦细芤迟。小便已,洒洒然毛耸。手足逆冷。小有劳,身即热,口开,前板齿燥。若发其汗,则恶寒甚;加温铖,则发热甚;数下之,则淋甚。

25. A person with sunstroke of Initial yang type may have a fever, chillphobia, generalized heaviness and pain, a chordal, thin, hollow, and slow pulse, a shivering sensation after urination, adverse chilling of the limbs, development of fever upon slight physical exertion, gasping, dry front teeth, violent chill phobia when perspiring, severe fever upon treatment with warm needles; and serious urinary dripping upon frequent purgation.

第二十六节　太阳中热者,暍是也。汗出恶寒,身热而渴,白虎加人参汤主之。
白虎加人参汤方:知母六两,石膏一斤(碎),甘草二两,粳米六合,人参三两。
上五味,以水一斗,煮米熟汤成,去滓,温服一升,日三服。

26. Heatstroke (Re), a Initial yang disease, manifests sweating, chillphobia, generalized fever, and thirst. Bai-hu-jia-ren-sheng-tang (Ginseng and Gypsum Combination) is the primary treatment.

6 liang anemarrhena

6 ge non-glutinous rice

16 liang smashed gypsum

3 liang ginseng

2 liang licorice

Cook the ingredients in 10 sheng of water until the rice is well done. Discard the dregs. One sheng of the decoction is taken warmed three times a day.

第二十七节　太阳中暍,身热疼重,而脉微弱,此以夏月伤冷水,水行皮中所致也。一物瓜蒂汤主之。
一物瓜蒂汤方:瓜蒂二十个。
上剉,以水一升,煮取五合,去滓,顿服。

27. Heatstroke with generalized fever, aching and heaviness, and a minute and weak pulse occurs when cool water along with summer heat injures the body by water vapor moving about in the skin. yi-wu-gua-di-tang (Melon Pedicel One Herb Combination) is the principal treatment for this greater yang diseases.

20 pcs. melon pedicels

Shred the pedicels and decoct them in 1 sheng of water until 0.5 sheng remains. Discard the dregs. The decoction is taken in one draft.

百合狐惑阴阳毒病脉证治第三

III.

On Pulse Syndrome Complex and Treatment of Bai He, Hu Huo, and Yin Yang Du Disease

第一节　论曰:百合病者,百脉一宗,悉致其病也。意欲食复不能食,常默默,欲卧不能卧,欲行不能行,欲饮食,或有美时,或有不用闻食臭时,如寒无寒,如热无热,口苦,小便赤,诸药不能治,得药则剧吐利,如有神灵者,身形如和,其脉微数。每溺时头痛者,六十日乃愈;若溺时头不痛,淅然者,四十日愈;若溺快然,但头眩者,二十日愈。其证或未病而预见,或病四五日而出,或病二十日或一月微见者,各随证治之。

1. The Classic states: Bai he is a disease characterized by general malaisea desire but inability to eat, talk, lie down, or walk. The patient often appears quiescent. Sometimes he has an appetite, sometimes not. He feels cold but has no chills or else feels hot but has no fever. A bitter taste invades his mouth and his urine flows red. No drug can cure him because severe vomiting and dysentery occur upon ingestion of drugs. It seems as though a certain spirit has possessed him although he appears to be normal except for a minute and quick pulse. If his head aches when he urinates, it means he will recover in sixty days. If instead he feels chilled on urination, he will recover in forty days. If when he urinates profusely he experiences vertigo, he will recover in twenty days. The conformation of the disease may be observed even before the appearance of the disease, or four to five days after the appearance of the disease, or twenty days or even one month later. It is treated according to the individual's condition and conformation.

第二节　百合病,发汗后者,百合知母汤主之。
百合知母汤方:百合七枚(擘),知母三两(切)。
上先以水洗百合,渍一宿,当白沫出,去其水,更以泉水二升,煎取一升,去滓;别以泉水二升煎知母,取一升,去滓;后合和,煎取一升五合,分温再服。

2. A patient with Bai he who has erroneously received treatment by the sweating method should

be treated principally with Bai-he-zhi-mu-tang (Lily and Anemarrhena Combination).

7 pcs. mashed lily corms   3 liang cut anemarrhena

Wash and soak the lily corms overnight in water. When white froth appears, discard the water and decoct the corms in 2 sheng of spring water until 1 sheng remains. Meanwhile decoct anemarrhena in another 2 sheng of spring water until 1 sheng remains. After discarding the dregs, combine the two decoctions and boil them down to 1.5 sheng. The decoction is taken warmed in divided portions.

第三节　百合病下之后者,滑石代赭汤主之。

滑石代赭汤方:百合七枚(擘),滑石三两(碎,绵裹),代赭石如弹丸大一枚(碎,绵裹)。

上先以水洗百合,渍一宿,当白沫出,去其水,更以泉水二升,煎取一升,去滓;别以泉水二升煎滑石、代赭,取一升,去滓,后合和重煎,取一升五合,分温服。

3. A patient with Bai he mistreated with purgatives should be given principally Hua-shi-dai-zhe-tang (Talc and Hematite Combination).

7 pcs. mashed lily corms   1 pc. bullet-sized ball of hematite, mashed
3 liang mashed talc wrapped in linen   and wrapped in linen

Wash and soak the lily corms in water until white froth appears. Discard the water and decoct the corms in 2 sheng of spring water until 1 sheng remains. At the same time, decoct the other two ingredients in 2 sheng of spring water until 1 sheng remains. After discarding the dregs combine the decoctions and reboil them down to 1.5 sheng. Tile decoction is divided into portions and taken warmed.

第四节　百合病,吐之后者,用后方(百合鸡子汤)主之。

百合鸡子汤方:百合七枚(擘),鸡子黄一枚。

上先以水洗百合,渍一宿,当白沫出,去其水,更以泉水二升,煎取一升,去滓,内鸡子黄,搅匀,煎五分,温服。

4. Bai he erroneously treated by the vomiting method requires principally Bai-he-ji-zhi-tang (Lily and Yolk Combination).

7 pcs. mashed lily corms   1 pcs. egg yolk

Prepare the lily as indicated in the preceding formulas. In the final decoction, add the egg yoke and decoct the two ingredients for 5 minutes. The solution is taken warm.

第五节　百合病,不经吐、下、发汗,病形如初者,百合地黄汤主之。

百合地黄汤方:百合七枚(擘),生地黄汁一升。

上以水洗百合,渍一宿,当白沫出,去其水,更以泉水二升,煎取一升,去滓,内地黄汁,煎取一升五合,分温再服。中病,勿更服。大便当如漆。

5. Bai he disease, not treated with the vomiting, purgation, or sweating methods, that lingers in the same condition as in the beginning needs Bai-he-di-huang-tang(Lily and Rehmannia Combination).

7 pcs. mashed lily corms   1 sheng raw rehmannia juice

Prepare the lily corms as indicated in the preceding formulas. In the final decoction, add the raw rehmannia juice, and reboil the mixed solution down to 1.5 sheng. Divide the decoction into two portions and take each portion warmed. Once the drug takes effect, it should be suspended. It must be noted that during administration of the drug, the patient's stools always appear as dark as a black varnish.

第六节　百合病,一月不解,变成渴者,百合洗方主之。
百合洗方:上以百合一升,以水一斗,渍之一宿,以洗身。洗已,食煮饼,勿以盐豉也。

6. A patient with bai he disease that has lasted for one month without alleviation will experience thirst as a major symptom. Bai-he-xi-fang (Lily Wash) is the principal treatment.

1 sheng lily corms   10 sheng water

Soak the lily corms in the water overnight and have the patient wash himself with the solution. After washing he should eat wheat cakes and avoid salt and soya bean relish.

第七节　百合病,渴不差者,用后方(栝蒌牡蛎散)主之。
栝蒌牡蛎散方:栝蒌根、牡蛎(熬)等分。上为细末,饮服方寸匕,日三服。

7. When Bai he with thirst persists, the principal treatment is Gua-lou-mu-li-san (Trichosanthes and Oyster Shell Formula).

trichosanthes root   stewed oyster shell

equal amounts of each

Grind the drugs in equal amounts into powder. Take one fang cunbi (1 gram) of the powder with water three times a day.

第八节　百合病变发热者,百合滑石散主之。
百合滑石散方:百合一两(炙),滑石二两(一作三两)。
上为散,饮服方寸匕,日三服。当微利者,止服,热则除。

8. A patient with Bai he disease who develops a fever should be treated with Bai-he-hua-shi-san (Lily and Talc Formula).

1 liang baked lily corm   2 liang talc

Pound the drugs into powder. Take one fangcunbi (1 gram) with water, three times a day. When slight diarrhea appears, stop taking the drug, as Heat has been eliminated.

第九节　百合病见于阴者,以阳法救之;见于阳者,以阴法救之。见阳攻阴,复发其汗,此为逆;见阴攻阳,乃复下之,此亦为逆。

9. Bai he disease with yin symptoms should be treated with the yang method (nourishing and warming the yang) and vice versa. It is adverse treatment to attack the yin and induce perspiration in the presence of yang symptoms. Attacking yang followed by purgation in the presence of yin symptoms is also adverse treatment.

第十节　狐惑之为病,状如伤寒,默默欲眠,目不得闭,卧起不安,蚀于喉为惑,蚀于阴为狐,不欲饮食,恶闻食臭,其面目乍赤、乍黑、乍白,蚀于上部则声喝,甘草泻心汤主之。

甘草泻心汤方:甘草四两(炙),黄芩、人参、干姜各三两,黄连一两,大枣十二枚(擘),半夏半升。

上七味,水一斗,煮取六升,去滓再煎,温服一升,日三服。

10. Hu huo resembles shang han disease in that the patient looks moribund and is somnolent and unable to close his eyes and so restless that he continually lies down and gets up. An ulcer in the larynx is Huo disease while an ulcer on the pudendum or the anus is Hu disease. The patient, repelled by the odor of food, will be anorexic, and his facial color will vary from red to dark to pale. If ulceration develops in the upper part of the body, hoarseness occurs. The condition should principally be treated with Gan-cao-xie-xin-tang (Pinellia and Licorice Combination).

4 liang baked licorice   1 liang coptis

3 liang scute   12 pcs. jujube fruits mashed

3 liang ginseng   0.5 sheng pinellia

3 liang dried ginger

Decoct the ingredients with 10 sheng of water until 6 sheng remains. Discard the dregs and decoct the solution again until 3 sheng remains. One sheng warmed is taken three times daily.

第十一节　蚀于下部则咽干,苦参汤洗之。蚀于肛者,雄黄熏之。

雄黄:上一味为末,筒瓦二枚合之,烧,向肛熏之。

苦参汤方:苦参一升,以水一斗,煎取七升,去滓,熏洗,日三服。

11. Ulceration on the pudendum is preceded by pharyngeal dryness. The pudendum should be washed with Ku-sheng-tang(Sophora Wash); ulceration on the anus should be treated with Xiong-

huang (realgar) fumigation.

Sophora Wash:

1 sheng sophora   10 sheng water

Decoct 1 sheng of sophora in 10 sheng of water until 7 sheng remains and discard the dregs.
After fumigating the genitals, wash them with the decoction three times daily.

Realgar Fumigation:

Place ground realgar in a cylinder formed by two semicylindrical rooftiles. Place the tiles on a
fire in order to produce fumes, and direct the fumes toward the anus.

第十二节　病者脉数,无热,微烦,默默但欲卧,汗出,初得之三四日,目赤如鸠眼;七
八日,目四眦黑。若能食者,脓已成也,赤豆当归散主之。

赤豆当归散方:赤小豆三升(浸令芽出,曝干),当归三两。

上二味,杵为散,浆水服方寸匕,日三服。

12. If a patient with anal ulceration has a quick pulse, no fever, and mild vexation; remains
silent and wants to stay in bed; perspires heavily and has hyperemia of the eyes (their being as red
as a dove's eyes) after three or four days of the disease; has black discoloration at the four corners
of the eyes after sevenor eight days of the disease; and can ingest food, it indicates suppuration has
developed. The condition should be principally treated with Chi-dou-dang-gui-san (Phaseolus and
Dang-gui Formula).

3 sheng phaseolus soaked in water to induce sprouting, then dried in the sun

3 liang dang-gui

Pound the two ingredients into powder. One fangcunbi of the powder mixed in soil water is tak-
en three times daily.

第十三节　阳毒之为病,面赤斑斑如锦纹,咽喉痛,唾脓血。五日可治,七日不可治,
升麻鳖甲汤主之。

阴毒之为病,面目青,身痛如被杖,咽喉痛。五日可治,七日不可治,升麻鳖甲汤去雄
黄、蜀椒主之。

升麻鳖甲汤方:升麻二两,当归一两,蜀椒(炒去汗)一两,甘草二两,雄黄半两(研),
鳖甲手指大一片(炙)。上六味,以水四升,煮取一升,顿服之,老小再服,取汗。

13. Yang du manifests silky red macules on the face, a sore throat, and expectoration of purulent blood; it is curable if treated within five days, but incurable beyond seven days of onset. Treatment calls for Sheng-ma-bie-jia-tang (Cimicifuga and Tortoise Shell Combination). Yin du exhibits
a bluish discoloration of the face and in the whites of the eyes, generalized aching (as if beaten with
a stick), and a sore throat.

It is curable within five days and incurable beyond seven days. Principal treatment calls for Sheng-ma-bie-jia-tang-qu-xiong-huang-shu-jiao (Cimicifuga and Tortoise Shell Combination, excluding realgar and zanthoxylum).

2 liang cimicifuga   2 liang licorice

1 liang dang-gui   0.5 liang ground realgar

1 liang zanthoxylum fried to expel the oil   1 finger-like portion of baked tortoise shell

Decoct the six ingredients in 4 sheng of water until the volume is reduced to 1 sheng. The decoction induces sweating when taken all in one draft by adults, or is divided into two portions with one portion taken twice a day by elderly or young patients.

疟病脉证并治第四

IV.

On Pulse Syndrome Complex and Treatment of Malaria

第一节 师曰:疟脉自弦,弦数者多热,弦迟者多寒。弦小紧者下之差,弦迟者可温之,弦紧者可发汗、针灸也,浮大者可吐之,弦数者风发也,以饮食消息止之。

1. The master said:"A patient with malaria characteristically has a chordal pulse. A chordal, quick pulse often accompanies a fever while a chordal, slow pulse goes with chills. A patient with a chordal, thin, and tense pulse requires purging;one with a chordal and slow pulse, warming; one with a chordal and tense pulse, sweating, acupuncture, or moxibustion; and one with a floating and big pulse, emesis. A chordal and quick pulse signifies a fever due to 'wind evil'. An appropriate diet according to the condition eliminates the fever.

第二节 病疟以月一日发,当以十五日愈;设不差,当月尽解;如其不差,当如何? 师曰:此结为症瘕,名曰疟母,急治之,宜鳖甲煎丸。

鳖甲煎丸方:鳖甲十二分(炙),乌扇三分(烧),黄芩三分,柴胡六分,鼠妇三分(熬),干姜三分,大黄三分,芍药五分,桂枝三分,葶苈一分(熬),石韦三分(去毛),厚朴三分,牡丹五分(去心),瞿麦二分,紫葳三分,半夏一分,人参一分,䗪虫五分(熬),阿胶三分(炙),蜂窝四分(炙),赤硝十二分,蜣蜋六分(熬),桃仁二分。

上二十三味,为末,取锻灶下灰一斗,清酒一斛五斗,浸灰,候酒尽一半,着鳖甲于中,煮令泛烂如胶漆,绞取汁,内诸药,煎为丸,如梧子大,空心服七丸,日三服。

2. The disciples asked:"Malaria occurring on the first day of the month, for example, usually will heal by the fifteenth day. If not, it ought to heal by the end of the month. What is wrong if it has not healed by then?"

The master answered:"An abdominal tumor known as Nue mu has developed if malaria does not go away. The doctor should treat the patient promptly with Bie-jia-jian-wan(Tortoise Shell Formula)."

12 fen baked tortoise shell	5 fen cored moutan
3 fen burnt belamcanda	2 fen dianthus
3 fen scute	3 fen decoma
3 fen bupleurum	1 fen pinellia
3 fen stewed porcellio scaber	1 fen ginseng
3 fen dried ginger	5 fen stewed eupolyphaga
3 fen rhubarb	3 fent baked gelatin
5 fen peony	4 fen baked hornets' and wasps' nests
3 fen cinnamon	12 fen red nitre
1 fen stewed lepidium	6 fen stewed scarab beetle
3 fen dehaired pyrrosia	2 fen persica seed
3 fen magnolia	

Grind all of the ingredients except the tortoise shell into powder. To prepare the tortoise shell, first soak 10 sheng of ashes from a forging furnace in 1 jin and 5 dou of clear wine. When the liquid has reduced by half, add the tortoise shell to the wine-ash mixture and cook until the shell becomes gelatinous. Strain the mixture. Mix the juice with the previously prepared powder and decoct again. Make the resultant paste into pills the size of a sterculia seed. Seven pills are taken three times daily on an empty stomach.

第三节　师曰:阴气孤绝,阳气独发,则热而少气烦冤,手足热而欲呕,名曰瘅疟。若但热不寒者,邪气内藏于心,外舍分肉之间,令人消烁脱肉。

3. The master said: "When yin Qi is isolated and depleted, yang Qi flourishes causing fever, diminished Qi, vexation and melancholy, feverish extremities, and a tendency to vomit. The condition is known as dan nue. If the patient has only a fever without chills, toxic Qi has become lodged in the heart or in the exterior between the muscles causing emaciation."

第四节　温疟者,其脉如平,身无寒但热,骨节疼烦,时呕,白虎加桂枝汤主之。
白虎加桂枝汤方:知母六两,甘草二两(炙),石膏一斤,粳米二合,桂枝(去皮)三两。
上剉每五钱,水一盏半,煎至八分,去滓,温服,汗出愈。

4. Wen nue (Warm malaria) manifests a normal pulse, absence of chilis, generalized fever, arthralgia, vexation, and frequent vomiting. It is treated principally with Bai-hu-jia-gui-zhi-tang (Cinnamon and Gypsum Combination).

6 liang anemarrhena	2 ge non-glutinous rice
2 liang baked licorice	3 liang cinnamon with the bark removed
16 liang gypsum	

Pound the drugs. Divide into five qian doses. Stew each dose in one and a half cups of water until eight fen remain. Filter the decoction and serve warm. When perspiration is induced, syndrome disappears as well.

第五节　疟多寒者,名曰牝疟,蜀漆散主之。

蜀漆散方:蜀漆(洗去腥)、云母(烧二日夜),龙骨等分。

上三味,杵为散,未发前以浆水服半钱。

5. A malarial disease with more chills than fever is called Pin nue (female malaria); Shu-qi-san (Dichroa Sprout and Mica Formula) is the principal treatment.

Dichroa sprout washed to remove the fishy odor

Mica baked for two days and nights

Dragon bone

equal amounts of each.

Pound the ingredients into powder. 0.5 qian of the powder mixed with soil water is taken before a seizure. For wen nue(warm malaria), incorporate an additional 0.5 fen of dichroa, and take one liang-coinful of the powder upon seizure.

第六节　附《外台秘要》方。

6. Three other formulas from the *Wai Tai Mi Yao* also treat malaria.

牡蛎汤:治牝疟。牡蛎四两(熬),麻黄四两(去节),甘草二两,蜀漆三两。

上四味,以水八升,先煮蜀漆、麻黄,去上沫,得六升,内诸药,煮取二升,温服一升,若吐,则勿更服。

Mu-li-tang (Oyster Shell Combination) treats pin nue (male malaria).

4 liang stewed oyster shell	2 liang licorice
4 liang denuded mahuang	3 liang dichroa

First decoct dichroa and mahuang with 8 sheng of water; then skim off the floating foam and boil until 6 sheng remains; add the other herbs and continue decocting until 2 sheng remains. One sheng warmed is taken. If vomiting occurs suspend taking of the formula.

柴胡去半夏加栝蒌根汤:治疟病发渴者,亦治劳疟。

柴胡八两,人参、黄芩、甘草各三两,栝蒌根四两,生姜二两,大枣十二枚。

上七味,以水一斗二升,煮取六升,去滓,再煎,取三升,温服一升,日二服。

Chai-hu-qu-ban-xia-jia-gua-lou-gen-tang (Bupleurum and Trichosanthes Root Combination) treats malaria with thirst and consumptive malaria.

8 liang bupleurum	4 liang trichosanthes root
3 liang ginseng	2 liang flesh ginger
3 liang scute	12 pcs. jujube fruits
3 liang licorice	

Decoct the herbs with 12 sheng of water until 6 sheng remains; remove the dregs and decoct again until 3 sheng remains. One sheng is taken warmed twice daily.

柴胡桂姜汤：治疟寒多微有热，或但寒不热。

柴胡半斤，桂枝三两(去皮)，干姜二两，栝蒌根四两，黄芩三两，牡蛎三两(熬)，甘草二两(炙)。

上七味，以水一斗二升，煮取六升，去滓，再煎，取三升，温服一升，日三服。初服微烦，复服汗出便愈。

Chai-hu-gui-jiang-tang (Bupleurum, Cinnamon, and Ginger Combination) treats malaria with chills and a mild fever or with chills and no fever.

8 liang bupleurum	4 liang trichosanthes
3 liang cinnamon stripped of the coarse outer skin	3 liang scute
	3 liang stewed oyster shell
2 liang dried ginger	2 liang baked licorice

Place the ingredients in 12 sheng of water and decoct until 6 sheng remains; remove the dregs and decoct again until 3 sheng remains. One sheng warmed is taken three times daily. After administration of the first dose, the patient may feel slightly vexed, but he will recover after perspiring has been induced by the subsequent administrations.

中风历节病脉证并治第五

V.

On Pulse Syndrome Complex and Treatment of Zhong Feng(Apoplexy) and Li Jie(Acute Arthritis)

第一节　夫风之为病,当半身不遂,或但臂不遂者,此为痹。脉微而数,中风使然。

1. Disease brought on by pathogenetic Wind will cause hemiplegia. When a patient cannot move one or both arms freely, it is a case of Bi syndrome with feeble-speedy pulse caused by pathogenetic Wind, known in Chinese as zhong feng (windstroke or apoplexy).

第二节　寸口脉浮而紧,紧则为寒,浮则为虚;寒虚相搏,邪在皮肤;浮者血虚,络脉空虚,贼邪不泄,或左或右,邪气反缓,正气即急,正气引邪,㖞僻不遂。邪在于络,肌肤不仁;邪在于经,即重不胜;邪入于腑,即不识人;邪入于脏,舌即难言,口吐涎。

侯氏黑散:治大风四肢烦重,心中恶寒不足者。

菊花四十分,白术十分,细辛三分,茯苓三分,牡蛎三分,桔梗八分,防风十分,人参三分,矾石三分,黄芩五分(一本作三分),当归三分,干姜三分,芎䓖三分,桂枝三分。

上十四味,杵为散,酒服方寸匕,日一服,初服二十日,温酒调服,禁一切鱼肉大蒜,常宜冷食,六十日止,即药积在腹中不下也。热食即下矣,冷食自能助药力。

2. A floating and tense pulse at the cun site, "floating" signifying weakness and "tense" chills, means that chills and weakness are in interaction with each other and the "evil" has lodged in the skin. A floating pulse portends blood weakness and meridian emptiness attributable to accumulated "wind evil" and its subsequent stagnation in either the left or the right side of the body. Thus unbalanced Qi slows and normal Qi accelerates drawing the unbalanced Qi. Skewing of the mouth and paralysis result.

Evil lodged in the superficial meridians (luo) causes skin numbness; evil in the inner meridians (jing) causes heaviness and impaired movement of the extremities. Evil in the hollow viscera (gallbladder, stomach, small intestines, large intestines, and urinary bladder) causes insanity while evil in the solid viscera (heart, liver, spleen, lungs, and kidneys) makes the tongue unable to articulate and causes slobbering.

Hou-shi-hei-san (Chrysanthemum and Siler Formula) treats severe wind disease causing annoying heaviness in the arms and legs and mild chillphobia in the heart.

40 fen chrysanthemum	3 fen ginseng
10 fen atractylodes	3 fen alum
3 fen asarum	5 fen scute
3 fen hoelen	3 fen tang-kuei
3 fen oyster shell	3 fen dried ginger
8 fen platycodon	3 fen cnidium
10 fen siler	3 fen cinnamon

Pound the drugs into powder. Take one fangcunbi with wine per dose once a day. During the first twenty days, take with warm wine. Avoid eating fish, meat, garlic, and eat cold food when possible. Continue for sixty days. Drugs will accumulate in the abdomen. If hot meals are taken, drugs will not remain in the abdomen. Cold food can increase the efficacy of the drugs.

第三节　寸口脉迟而缓,迟则为寒,缓则为虚,营缓则为亡血,卫缓则为中风。邪气中经,则身痒而瘾疹;心气不足,邪气入中,则胸满而短气。

3. A slow and moderate pulse on the cun site portends chills, as indicated by the "slow" character, and weakness, as indicated by the "moderate" character. A weak ying Qi (blood system) follows a loss of blood. When wei (protective system) weakens, zhong feng (windstroke or apoplexy) occurs. When evil Qi affects the inner meridians, generalized pruritus and urticaria result. If heart Qi is insufficient and the evil Qi has invaded the interior, the patient experiences chest distention and gasping.

风引汤:除热瘫痫。

大黄、干姜、龙骨各四两,桂枝三两,甘草、牡蛎各二两,寒水石、滑石、赤石脂、白石脂、紫石英、石膏各六两。

上十二味,杵,粗筛,以韦囊盛之,取三指撮,井花水三升,煮三沸,温服一升。

Feng-yin-tang (Rhubarb and Dragon Bone Combination) eliminates paralysis and convulsions caused by fever.

4 liang rhubarb	6 liang gypsum and calcite
4 liang dried ginger	6 liang talc
4 liang dragon bone	6 liang hematite
3 liang cinnamon	6 liang kaolin

2 liang licorice

6 liang amethyst

2 liang oyster shell

6 liang gypsum

Pulverize the ingredients by pounding and put them through a crude screen; store the powder in a leather bag. Take a quantity of the powder by pinching with three fingers: thumb, forefinger, and middle finger, decoct and boil with 3 sheng of well water for a short while. One sheng is taken warmed.

防己地黄汤：治病如狂状，妄行，独语不休，无寒热，其脉浮。

防己一钱，桂枝三钱，防风三钱，甘草二钱。

上四味，以酒一杯，浸之一宿，绞取汁，生地黄二斤咬咀，蒸之如斗米饭久，以铜器盛其汁，更绞地黄汁，和，分再服。

For manic, irrational behavior, for example, incessant monologues, in people without chills or fever who have a buoyant pulse prescribe Fang-ji-di-huang-tang (Stephania and Rehmannia Combination).

10 fen stephania

30 fen siler

30 fen cinnamon

10 fen licorice

Soak the four herbs in one glass of wine overnight and strain the juice. Meanwhile shred 2 catties of raw rehmannia and steam for as long as it takes to cook 10 sheng of rice. Collect the juice in a copper vessel and strain the rehmannia to obtain more juice. Collect all the juices and mix with the first wine juice. Divide the mixture into two portions. Each portion is taken twice a day.

头风摩散方：

大附子一枚(炮)，盐等分。

上二味，为散，沐了，以方寸匕，已摩"疾"上，令药力行。

Tou-feng-mo-san (Aconite and Salt Formula)

1 large baked aconite root

table salt

equal amounts of each

Pound the two ingredients to powder. After the patient has taken a bath, rub the powder onto the lesion. This accelerates the drug effect.

第四节　寸口脉沉而弱，沉即主骨，弱即主筋，沉即为肾，弱即为肝。汗出入水中，如水伤心，历节黄汗出，故曰历节。

4. Pulse at Cunkou is deep-weak. Deep pulse indicates the diseaseis affecting the bones, and

is also a manifestation of a Kidney disease. Weak pulse indicates disease in tendons, and is also a manifestation of a Liver disease. When the patient is immersed in water when sweating all over, the pathogenetic Water will affect his Heart. Acute arthritis will occur with yellowish sweat. The condition is known as lijie(polyarthritis).

第五节　趺阳脉浮而滑,滑则谷气实,浮则汗自出。

5. When the pulse on the fu yang (foot tarsus) site is floating and slippery, the slipperiness indicates full gastric vitality and the floating, spontaneous sweating.

第六节　少阴脉浮而弱,弱则血不足,浮则为风,风血相搏,即疼痛如掣。

6. A lesser yin pulse that is floating and weak portends blood deficiency, as indicated by the weakness, and wind evil, as indicated by the floating. Interaction between wind evil and blood causes severe pain.

第七节　盛人脉涩小,短气,自汗出,历节痛,不可屈伸,此皆饮酒汗出当风所致。

7. If a stout individual is short of breath, has a harsh and thin pulse, and spontaneous sweating and severe joint pain that limits flexion and extension, he is suffering from drinking of liquor and perspiring while in a draft.

第八节　诸肢节疼痛,身体尪羸,脚肿如脱,头眩短气,温温欲吐,桂枝芍药知母汤主之。

桂枝芍药知母汤方:桂枝四两,芍药三两,甘草二两,麻黄二两,生姜五两,白术五两,知母四两,防风四两,附子二枚(一本作二两)(炮)。

上九味,以水七升,煮取二升,温服七合,日三服。

8. Joint pain in the extremeties, emaciation, foot edema that is so severe the feet feel detached, vertigo, gasping, and nausea require the principal treatment of Gui-zhi-shao-yao-zhi-mu-tang (Cinnamon and Anemarrhena Combination).

4 liang cinnamon	5 liang atractylodes
3 liang peony	4 liang anemarrhena
2 liang licorice	4 liang siler
2 liang mahuang	2 liang baked aconite
5 liang fresh ginger	

Decoct the ingredients in 7 sheng of water until 2 sheng remains. 0.7 sheng warmed is taken three times daily.

第九节　味酸则伤筋,筋伤则缓,名曰泄。咸则伤骨,骨伤则痿,名曰枯。枯泄相搏,名曰断泄。营气不通,卫不独行,营卫俱微,三焦无所御,四属断绝,身体羸瘦,独足肿大,黄汗出,胫冷。假令发热,便为历节也。

9. The excessive eating of sour food injures the muscles causing them to lose tone. This condition is known as xie(wasting). Ingestion of excessive salt injures the bones causing paralysis. This condition is known as ku (withering). Interaction between wasting and withering is known as duan xie (exhaustion), a condition in which blood and Qi are not circulating and wei (protective system) fails. With blood and wei weakened, primordial Qi fails to reach the three warmers, the circulation of qi and blood in the arms and legs is interrupted, the body becomes emaciated, the feet swell, and yellow sweat and tibial chills occur. In the presence of fever, the condition is called li jie (polyarthritis).

第十节　病历节不可屈伸,疼痛,乌头汤主之。
乌头汤方：治脚气疼痛,不可屈伸。
麻黄、芍药、黄芪各三两, 甘草二两(炙),川乌五枚(㕮咀,以蜜二升,煎取一升,即出乌头)。
上五味,㕮咀四味,以水三升,煮取一升,去滓,内蜜煎中,更煎之,服七合。不知,尽服之。

10. Wu-tou-tang (Wu-tou Combination) principally treats arthritis so painful that the patient is unable to flex or extend his limbs.

3 liang mahuang	5 pcs. wu-tou roots shredded (decocted with 2
3 liang peony	sheng of honey until 1 sheng remains; the wu-
3 liang astragalus	tou is then discarded)
3 liang baked licorice	

Shred the first four ingredients and decoct them in 3 sheng of water until 1 sheng remains. Discard the dregs and add the honey solution and decoct again. A dose of 0.7 sheng is taken. If nothing happens, the remainder is taken.

第十一节　乌头汤方：治脚气疼痛,不可屈伸。
麻黄、芍药、黄芪各三两,甘草三两(炙),川乌五枚(㕮咀,以蜜二升,煎取一升,即出乌头)。
右五味,㕮咀四味,以水三升,煮取一升,去滓,内蜜煎中,更煎之,服七合。不知,尽服之。

11. Wu-tou-tang (Wu-tou Combination) treats foot Qi (beriberi) ache so painful that the patient is unable to flex and extend his feet. The composition, preparation, and administration of the formula are indicated in the preceding article. Six other formulas also effective in treating the above mentioned conditions follow.

矾石汤：治脚气冲心。矾石二两。
上一味，以浆水一斗五升，煎三五沸，浸脚良。

Fan-shi-tang (Alum Combination)
2 liang alum
Decoct the alum in 15 sheng of soil water until it boils. Let it cool a little, then reboil. Repeat the boiling three to five times. Soak the feet in the decoction. It is good for treating foot qi flushing toward the heart.

续命汤：治中风痱，身体不能自收持，口不能言，冒昧不知痛处，或拘急不得转侧。
麻黄、桂枝、当归、人参、石膏、干姜、甘草各三两，芎䓖一两，杏仁四十枚。
上九味，以水一斗，煮取四升，温服一升，当小汗，薄覆脊，凭几坐，汗出则愈，不汗，更服。无所禁，勿当风。并治但伏不得卧，咳逆上气，面目浮肿。

Mahuang and Ginseng Combination treats wind-paralysis (rheumatism) in which the patient is unable to control his body or speech. He feels dull, not knowing the aching areas, or has spasms so severe that he cannot turn himself over.

Xu-ming-tang (Mahuang and Ginseng Combination)

3 liang mahuang	3 liang dried ginger
3 liang cinnamon	3 liang licorice
3 liang tang-kuei	1 liang cnidium
3 liang ginseng	40 pcs. apricot seeds
3 liang gypsum	

Decoct the ingredients in 10 sheng of water until 4 sheng remains: one sheng is taken warmed. The patient will perspire lightly so he or she should be wrapped in a thin cloth and seatedat a table. As the sweat cleanses, he will recover. If no perspiring occurs, another dose is taken. Nothing is contraindicated except that the patient should avoid drafts. The formula also helps those who can only lie in a prone but not a supine position and who have a cough with flushing up of qi and edema of the face and eyes.

三黄汤：治中风手足拘急，百节疼痛，烦热心乱，恶寒，经日不欲饮食。

麻黄五分,独活四分,细辛二分,黄芪二分,黄芩三分。

上五味,以水六升,煮取二升,分温三服,一服小汗,二服大汗。心热加大黄二分,腹满加枳实一枚,气逆加人参三分,悸加牡蛎三分,渴加栝蒌根三分,先有寒加附子一枚。

San-huang-tang（Mahuang, Astragalus and Scute Combination）

5 fen mahuang	2 fen astragalus
4 fen duhuo	3 fen scute
2 fen asarum	

Decoct the ingredients in 6 sheng of water until 2 sheng remains, then divide into three portions. Each portion is taken warmed. The first dose will cause mild perspiring and the second dose, great perspiring. For cardiac heat, add 2 fen of rhubarb; for abdominal distention, one fruit of zhishi; for Qi flushing, 3 fen of ginseng; for palpitation, 3 fen of oyster shell; for thirst, 3 fen of trichosanthes; and for chills preceding other symptoms, one aconite root.

Mahuang, Astragalus, and Scute Combination treats wind stroke with spasms in the hands and feet, arthralgia, an annoying fever and disturbed mind, chillphobia, and day-long loss of appetite.

术附汤:治风虚头重眩,苦极,不知食味,暖肌补中,益精气。

白术二两,甘草一两(炙),附子一枚半(炮去皮)。

上三味,剉,每五钱匕,姜五片,枣一枚,水盏半,煎七成,去滓,温服。

Shu-fu-tang（White Atractylodes and Aconite Combination）

2 liang white atractylodes	1.5 pcs. baked aconite roots with the outer
1 liang baked licorice	skin removed

Cut the ingredients to fine particles; decoct one half-qian-coinful of the powder with 1.5 zhan of water together with five ginger slices and one jujube fruit until 0.7 zhan remains; remove the dregs; the decoction is taken warmed.

Atractylodes and Aconite Combination treats evil wind and bodily weakness that cause heavy head, vertigo, severe distress, and loss of taste. It warms the muscles, supplements the stomach, and enriches the sperm.

崔氏八味丸:治脚气上入,少腹不仁。

干地黄八两,山茱萸、薯蓣各四两,泽泻、茯苓、牡丹皮各三两,桂枝、附子(炮)各一两。

上八味,末之,炼蜜和丸梧子大。酒下十五丸,日再服。

Cui-shi-ba-wei-wan（Rehmannia Eight Formula）

8 liang dry rehmannia	3 liang hoelen

4 liang cornus   3 liang moutan

4 liang dioscorea   1 liang cinnamon

3 liang alisma   1 liang baked aconite

Pulverize the ingredients, then knead with honey and make into pills the size of asterculia seed. Fifteen pills are taken twice daily with wine.

Rehmannia Eight Formula treats foot Qi that flushes up into the lower abdomen causing numbness.

越婢加术汤：治肉极，热则身体津脱，腠理开，汗大泄，厉风气，下焦脚弱。

麻黄六两，石膏半斤，生姜三两，甘草二两，白术四两，大枣十五枚。

上六味，以水六升，先煮麻黄去沫，内诸药，煮取三升，分温三服。恶风加附子一枚，炮。

Yue-pi-jia-shu-tang (Atractylodes Combination)

6 liang mahuang   2 liang licorice

8 liang gypsum   4 liang atractylodes

2 liang fresh ginger   15 pcs. jujube fruits

Decoct mahuang in 6 sheng of water, skim off the foam, add the other ingredients, and continue decoction until 3 sheng remains. Next discard the dregs and divide the decoction into three portions. Take each portion warmed. If the patient has anemophobia, add one baked aconite root.

Atractylodes Combination treats muscle exhaustion which in the presence of fever exhibits loss of body fluids, enlarged pores and muscular looseness, and profuse sweating. It also alleviates severe wind and weakness of the lower warmer and feet.

血痹虚劳病脉证并治第六

VI.

On Pulse Syndrome Complex and Treatment of Blood Paralysis and Weakness Fatigue

第一节　问曰:血痹病从何得之? 师曰:夫尊荣人骨弱肌肤盛,重因疲劳汗出,卧不时动摇,加被微风,遂得之。但以脉自微涩在寸口、关上小紧,宜针引阳气,令脉和紧去则愈。

1. The disciples asked: "What is the cause of blood paralysis?"

The master said: "Persons who live lives of leisure generally have weak bones and rich flesh and muscle. After working for a short period of time, they will feel tired and begin to sweat. When they lie in bed, they will toss and turn frequently. If they are exposed to a breeze at this time, they will suffer from arthralgia due to stagnation of Blood. The pulse will be feeble and hesitant and slender-tense at Inch and Bar. Acupuncture therapy can be adopted to stimulate Yang Vital Energy. When the tense pulse disappears and the pulse returns to normal, the patient is recovering."

第二节　血痹阴阳俱微,寸口关上微,尺中小紧,外证身体不仁,如风痹状,黄芪桂枝五物汤主之。

黄芪桂枝五物汤方:黄芪三两,芍药三两,桂枝三两,生姜六两,大枣十二枚。

上五味,以水六升,煮取二升,温服七合,日三服。

2. The patient suffering from "blood paralysis" with a minute pulse palpable both superficially and deeply on the cun and guan sites, a thin and tense pulse on the chi site, and an external conformation exhibiting generalized numbness like that of wind paralysis should be principally treated with Huang-qi-gui-zhi-wu-wu-tang (Astragalus and Cinnamon Five Herb Combination).

3 liang astragalus   6 liang fresh ginger

3 liang peony   12 pcs. jujube fruits

3 liang cinnamon

Decoct the ingredients in 6 sheng of water until 2 sheng remains. 0.7 sheng warmed is taken three times a day. A similar formula from another source also includes ginseng as an ingredient.

第三节　夫男子平人,脉大为劳,极虚亦为劳。

3．In men with a normal appearance, a big pulse portends weakness fatigue as does an extremely empty pulse.

第四节　男子面色薄者,主渴及亡血,卒喘悸,脉浮者,里虚也。

4．A pale complexion in men portends thirst and loss of blood. Paroxysmal asthma and cardiac palpitation together with a floating pulse portend internal weakness.

第五节　男子脉虚沉弦,无寒热,短气里急,小便不利,面色白,时目瞑,兼衄,少腹满,此为劳使之然。

5．The symptoms of weakness fatigue in men are an empty submerged, and chordal pulse, no chills and fever, shortness of breath, a feeling of urgent tension in the abdomen (like a need to defecate or urinate), oliguria, a pale complexion, frequent vertigo causing closure of eyes, nosebleeds, and lower abdominal distention.

第六节　劳之为病,其脉浮大,手足烦,春夏剧,秋冬瘥,阴寒精自出,酸削不能行。

6．Weakness fatigue exhibits a floating and big pulse, pudendal chills with spermatorrhea in men, aching and emaciated feet inhibiting walking, irritating fever in the limbs which exacerbates in the spring and summer and spontaneously dissipates in the autumn and winter.

第七节　男子脉浮弱而涩,为无子,精气清冷。

7．A floating, weak, and harsh pulse in a man means thin, chilly sperm and Qi, and sterility.

第八节　夫失精家,少腹弦急,阴头寒,目眩,发落,脉极虚芤迟,为清谷亡血,失精。脉得诸芤动微紧,男子失精,女子梦交,桂枝龙骨牡蛎汤主之。
　　桂枝龙骨牡蛎汤方:桂枝、芍药、生姜各三两,甘草二两,大枣十二枚,龙骨、牡蛎各三两。
　　上七味,以水七升,煮取三升,分温三服。

8．A man who loses semen without orgasm will have a tense and urgent sensation in the lower abdomen, chills in the glans of the penis, dizziness, loss of hair, and an extremely weak, hollow, and slow pulse. These symptoms accompany lientery, loss of blood, or spermatorrhea. In such cases the pulse is hollow, fluttering, minute, and tense. The man who has spermatorrhea and the women who dreams of sexual intercourse need Gui-zhi-long-gu-mu-li-tang (Cinnamon and Dragon Bone Combination).

3 liang cinnamon	12 pcs. jujube fruits
3 liang peony	3 liang dragon bone
3 liang fresh ginger	3 liang oyster shell
2 liang licorice	

Decoct the ingredients in 7 sheng of water until 3 sheng remains. It is taken warmed in three equal portions.

天雄散方：天雄三两(炮),白术八两,桂枝六两,龙骨三两。
上四味,杵为散,酒服半钱匕,日三服,不知,稍增之。

Another formula also treats this condition.
Tian-xiong-san (Aconite and Dragon Bone Formula)

3 liang baked aconite	6 liang cinnamon
8 liang atractylodes	3 liang dragon bone

Pound the drugs into powder. Take one half qianbi with wine three times a day. If not effective, increase the dosage slightly.

第九节　男子平人,脉虚弱细微者,喜盗汗也。

9. A man who appears normal but has an empty, weak, thin, and minute pulse will have night sweats readily.

第十节　人年五六十,其病脉大者,痹侠背行,若肠鸣,马刀侠瘿者,皆为劳得之。

10. A person in his fifties with a big pulse must have been afflicted by wind evil if he has a numb sensation along both sides of the spine, by internal chill if he has borborygmus, or by weak fever if tubercles have developed under the armpits or on the neck. All of these conditions are fatigue diseases.

第十一节　脉沉小迟,名脱气,其人疾行则喘喝,手足逆寒,腹满,甚则溏泄,食不消化也。

11. A submerged, thin, and slow pulse characterizes the condition known as tuo Qi (collapse

of Qi) in which the patient experiences shortness of breath when walking briskly, adverse chills in the arms and legs, and/or abdominal distention and even lientery owing to indigestion.

第十二节　脉弦而大,弦则为减,大则为芤,减则为寒,芤则为虚,虚寒相搏,此名为革。妇人则半产漏下,男子则亡血失精。

12. In a chordal and big pulse, "chordal" denotes deficiency and "big" hollowness; deficiency manifests through chills while hollowness indicates weakness. When weakness and chills spermatorrhea in men.

第十三节　虚劳里急,悸,衄,腹中痛,梦失精,四肢酸疼,手足烦热,咽干口燥,小建中汤主之。

小建中汤方：桂枝三两(去皮),甘草三两(炙),大枣十二枚,芍药六两,生姜三两,胶饴一升。

上六味,以水七升,煮取三升,去滓,内胶饴,更上微火消解,温服一升,日三服。

13. Weakness fatigue and internal cramps together with cardiac palpitation, nosebleeds, abdominal aches, nocturnal emission, soreness and aching in the extremities, fever in the limbs, and dry throat and mouth are primarily treated with Xiao-jian-zhong-tang (Minor Cinnamon and Peony Combination).

3 liang decorticated cinnamon	6 liang peony
3 liang baked licorice	3 liang fresh ginger
12 pcs. jujube fruits	1 sheng maltose

Decoct all the ingredients except the maltose in 7 sheng of water until 3 sheng remains; after discarding the dregs, add the maltose. Heat the contents on a mild fire to dissolve the maltose. One sheng of the warmed decoction is taken three times daily. A vomiting patient should not take this formula because its sweet taste will induce more vomiting.

第十四节　虚劳里急,诸不足,黄芪建中汤主之。

于小建中汤内加黄芪一两半,余依上法。气短胸满者加生姜;腹满者去枣,加茯苓一两半;及疗肺虚损不足,补气加半夏三两。

14. Weakness fatigue, internal cramps, and deficiencies of various types should be treated primarily with Huang-qi-jian-zhong-tang (Astragalus Combination).

To make Astragalus Combination, add 1.5 liang of astragalus to the preceding formula (Xiao-jian-zhong-tang) and prepare in the same way. For patients who are short of breath and have thoracic distention, add fresh ginger; for abdominal distention, exclude jujube fruits and add 1.5 liang of hoelen; for weakness injury of the lungs and for replenishing Qi, add 3 liang of pinellia.

第十五节　虚劳腰痛,少腹拘急,小便不利者,八味肾气丸主之。

肾气丸方：干地黄八两,山药、山茱萸各四两,泽泻、牡丹皮、茯苓各三两,桂枝、附子(炮)各一两。

上八味末之,炼蜜和丸梧桐子大,酒下十五丸,加至二十五丸,日再服。

15. A patient with weakness fatigue disease, lower back pain, lower abdominal cramping, and oliguria should primarily take Ba-wei-Shen-Qi-wan (Rehmannia Eight Formula).

8 liang dry rehmannia	3 liang moutan
4 liang dioscorea	3 liang hoelen
4 liang cornus	1 liang cinnamon
3 liang alisma	1 liang baked aconite

Pulverize the eight ingredients, knead with honey, and form into pills the size of a sterculia seed. Fifteen pills (increasing to twenty-five) are taken twice daily with wine.

第十六节　虚劳诸不足,风气百疾,薯蓣丸主之。

薯蓣丸方：薯蓣三十分、当归、桂枝、曲、干地黄、豆黄卷各十分,甘草二十八分,人参七分,芎劳、芍药、白术、麦门冬、杏仁各六分,柴胡、桔梗、茯苓各五分,阿胶七分,干姜三分,白蔹二分,防风六分,大枣百枚为膏。

上二十一味,末之,炼蜜和丸,如弹子大,空腹酒服一丸,一百丸为剂。

16. Conditions of weakness fatigue, various kinds of insufficiency, and "wind and Qi" diseases primarily require Shu-yu-wan (Dioscorea and Jujube Formula).

30 fen dioscorea	6 fen ophiopogon
10 fen danggui	6 fen apricot seed
10 fen cinnamon	5 fen bupleurum
10 fen yeast	5 fen platycodon
10 fen dry rehmannia	5 fen hoelen
10 fen bean sprouts	7 fen gelatin
28 fen licorice	3 fen dried ginger
7 fen gindeng	2 fen ampelopsis
6 fen cnidium	6 fen siler
6 fen peony	100 pcs. jujube fruits made into a paste
6 fen atractylodes	

Pulverize the ingredients, knead with honey, and form into pills the size of a bullet. One pill is taken with wine on an empty stomach. The recipe yields 100 pills.

第十七节　虚劳虚烦不得眠,酸枣仁汤主之。

酸枣仁汤方:酸枣仁二升,甘草一两,知母二两,茯苓二两,芎劳二两。

上五味,以水八升,煮酸枣仁,得六升,内诸药,煮取三升,分温三服。

17. Suan-zao-ren-tang (Zizyphus Combination) primarily treats weakness fatigue, and annoyance due to weakness which causes insomnia.

2 sheng zizyphus	2 liang hoelen
1 liang licorice	2 liang cnidium
2 liang anemarrhena	

Decoct the zizyphus in 8 sheng of water until 6 sheng remains; then add the other ingredients and decoct again until the solution is reduced to 3 sheng. The decoction is divided into three portions and taken warmed three times daily.

第十八节　五劳虚极羸瘦,腹满不能饮食,食伤、忧伤、饮伤、房室伤、饥伤、劳伤、经络营卫气伤,内有干血,肌肤甲错,两目黯黑。缓中补虚,大黄䗪虫丸主之。

大黄䗪虫丸方:大黄十分(蒸),黄芩二两,甘草三两,桃仁一升,杏仁一升,芍药四两,干地黄十两,干漆一两,虻虫一升,水蛭百枚,蛴螬一升,䗪虫半升。

上十二味,末之,炼蜜和丸小豆大,酒饮服五丸,日三服。

18. The formula Da-huang-zhe-chong-wan (Rhubarb and Eupolyphaga Formula) mollifies the stomach, strengthens weakness, and is the principal treatment for the following conditions: the five fatigues; extreme weakness that leads to emaciation; abdominal distention and anorexia; injuries caused by foods, worry, drinking, sexual excess, starvation, and overstraining; and injury of Qi in the meridians, the skin, and the viscera which results in blood aridity, coarse and scaly skin, and darkened eyes.

10 fen steamed rhubarb	10 liang dried rehmannia
2 liang scute	1 liang dried lacquer
3 liang licorice	100 pieces of leech
4 liang peony	1 sheng tabanus
1 sheng persica	1 sheng holotrichia
1 sheng apricot seed	0.5 sheng eupolyphaga

Pound the twelve ingredients into powder, knead with honey, and make into pills the size of a small bean. Nine pills with wine are taken three times a day.

Two other formulas also treat weakness fatigue.

《千金翼》炙甘草汤:治虚劳不足,汗出而闷,脉结悸,行动如常,不出百日,危急者十一日死。

甘草四两(炙),桂枝、生姜各三两,麦门冬半升,麻仁半升,人参、阿胶各二两,大枣三十枚,生地黄一升。

上九味,以酒七升,水八升,先煮八味,取三升,去滓,内胶消尽,温服一升,日三服。

Zhi-gan-cao-tang (Baked Licorice Combination), treats weakness fatigue, deficiencies, perspiring with depression, a knotty pulse, and cardiac palpitation in the presence of normal activity. Patients with these symptoms will die within one hundred days, or in critical cases, within eleven days.

4 liang baked licorice	2 liang ginseng
3 liang cinnamon	2 liang gelatin
3 liang fresh ginger	30 pcs. jujube fruits
0.5 sheng ophiopogon	16 liang fresh (raw) rehmanni
0.5 sheng cannabis seeds	

Decoct all ingredients except gelatin in 7 sheng of wine and 8 sheng of water until 3 sheng remains. After discarding the dregs, add gelatin, wait until it completely dissolves, and then take one sheng of the decoction warmed three times daily.

《肘后》獭肝散:治冷劳,又主瘵疰一门相染。

獭肝一具,炙干末之,水服方寸匕,日三服。

Lai-gan-san (Otter Liver Powder) treats chill fatigue or infectious wasting disease. Bake one otter liver until dry, then pulverize it. Take one fangcunbi along with water three times daily.

肺痿肺痈咳嗽上气病脉证治第七

VII.

On Pulse Syndrome Complex and Treatment of Pulmonary Asthenia, Pulmonary Abscess and Cough with Qi Adversity

第一节　问曰:热在上焦者,因咳为肺痿。肺痿之病,从何得之? 师曰:或从汗出,或从呕吐,或从消渴,小便利数,或从便难,又被快药下利,重亡津液,故得之。曰:寸口脉数,其人咳,口中反有浊唾涎沫者何? 师曰:为肺痿之病。若口中辟辟燥,咳即胸中隐隐痛,脉反滑数,此为肺痈,咳唾脓血。脉数虚者为肺痿,数实者为肺痈。

1. The disciples asked: "When pathogenetic Heat is present in the Upper Portion of Body Cavity, the patient will suffer from coughing, followed by pulmonary asthenia. What is the cause of pulmonary asthenia?"

The master said: "It occurs as a consequence of excessive sweating, excessive vomiting, diabetes with polyuria, or constipation that has been treated with strong purgatives which have exhausted the body fluids."

The disciples further queried: "Pulse is speedy at the Inch. The patient coughs with sputum and saliva in his mouth. Why is this?"

The master answered: "This is a case of pulmonary asthenia. If the patient's mouth is parched and dry, if he experiences pain in his chest when coughing, and if pulse is slippery-speedy, it is a case of pulmonary abscess. Pulmonary asthenia always has symptoms of coughing with bloody pus and speedy-deficient pulse; whereas pulse of a patient suffering pulmonary abscess is always speedy-excessive."

第二节　问曰:病咳逆,脉之,何以知此为肺痈? 当有脓血,吐之则死,其脉何类? 师曰:寸口脉微而数,微则为风,数则为热;微则汗出,数则恶寒。风中于卫,呼气不入;热过于营,吸而不出。风伤皮毛,热伤血脉。风舍于肺,其人则咳,口干喘满,咽燥不渴,多唾浊沫,时时振寒。热之所过,血为之凝滞,蓄结痈脓,吐如米粥。始萌可救,脓成则死。

2. The disciples asked: "When there is an adverse cough, how can one tell if there is a pulmonary abscess? With a fatal pulmonary abscess the patient expectorates purulent blood. What type of pulse does this disease manifest?"

The master said: "With pulmonary abscess the patient has a minute and quick pulse on the cun site. The minute characteristic signifies wind evil, and the quickness, fever; the former evidences perspiration and the latter chillphobia. If wind evil has merely invaded the surface, the patient exhales more than he inhales. As the condition progresses, however, and the fever evil enters the viscera, the patient inhales more than he exhales, because the fever combines with the blood thus hindering the release of air. Generally "wind" injures the skin and hair while fever injures the blood vessels. Wind trapped in the lungs causes coughing, dry mouth, asthma, chest distention, dry throat without thirst, expectoration of copious thick sputum, and frequent shivering. With fever the blood congeals and stagnates, developing into abscesses. The expectorated matter resembles rice gruel. The disease is curable in the early stages but fatal if pus develops."

第三节 上气面浮肿,肩息,其脉浮大,不治,又加下利尤甚。

3. Symptoms of the flushing of Qi, facial edema, hunched shoulders, and a floating and big pulse indicate a condition difficult to cure. If diarrhea is also present, the condition is even worse.

第四节 上气喘而燥者属肺张,欲作风水,发汗则愈。

4. Flushing of Qi together with asthma and agitation is a condition characteristic of lung distention and indicates a predisposition to wind-water disease. The sweating method cures the condition.

第五节 肺痿吐涎沫而不咳者,其人不渴,必遗尿,小便数,所以然者,以上虚不能制下故也。此为肺中冷,必眩,多涎唾,甘草干姜汤以温之。若服汤已渴者,属消渴。

甘草干姜汤方:甘草四两(炙),干姜二两(炮)。

上二味,以水三升,煮取一升五合,去滓,分温再服。

5. A patient suffering from pulmonary asthenia who slobbers but doesn't cough and has no thirst will definitely have urinary incontinence and polyuria. This is because the upper portion of body cavity is weak and unable to control the lower torso; hence the lungs become cold (because the upper portion of body cavity is weak and cold, yang Qi cannot ascend). Therefore, the patient will doubtlessly have vertigo and excess saliva. Treatment calls for warming with Gan-cao-gan-jiang-tang (Licorice and Ginger Combination). If the patient becomes thirsty after taking this drug, he has diabetes.

4 liang baked licorice   2 liang baked dried ginger

Shred and decoct the ingredients in 3 sheng of water until 1.5 sheng remains; discard the dregs. The decoction is divided into two equal portions. One portion warmed is taken twice a day.

第六节　咳而上气,喉中水鸡声,射干麻黄汤主之。

射干麻黄汤方:射干三两,麻黄四两,生姜四两,细辛、紫菀、款冬花各三两,五味子半升,大枣七枚,半夏(大者洗)八枚。

上九味,以水一斗二升,先煮麻黄两沸,去上沫,内诸药,煮取三升,分温三服。

6. Cough with flushing of Qi and a croaking sound in the throat should be treated principally with She-gan-ma-huang-tang (Belamcanda and Mahuang Combination).

3 liang belamcancia	3 liang tussilago
4 liang mahuang	0.5 sheng schizandra
4 liang fresh ginger	7 pcs. jujube fruits
3 liang asarum	8 pcs. large pinellia corms washed
3 liang aster	

First boil mahuang in 12 sheng of water and skim the resulting foam off. Add the other ingredients and decoct again until 3 sheng remains. The decoction is divided into three equal portions. One portion is taken warmed three times a day.

第七节　咳逆上气,时时吐浊,但坐不得眠,皂荚丸主之。

皂荚丸方:皂荚八两(刮去皮,用酥炙)。

上一味,末之,蜜丸梧子大,以枣膏和汤服三丸,日三夜一服。

7. A patient who coughs with a flushing up of Qi and frequent expectoration of thick sputum and who can sit up but cannot sleep should be treated primarily with Zao-jia-wan(Gleditsia Formula).

8 liang gleditsia with the outer skin scraped off, baked in butter.

Pulverize the gleditsia and knead with honey. Make into pills the size of a sterculia seed. Three pills boiled in water are taken with jujube paste three times a day and once at night.

第八节　咳而脉浮者,厚朴麻黄汤主之。

厚朴麻黄汤方:厚朴五两 麻黄四两,石膏如鸡子大,杏仁半升,半夏半升,干姜二两,细辛二两,小麦一升,五味子半升。

上九味,以水一斗二升,先煮小麦熟,去滓,内诸药,煮取三升,温服一升,日三服。

8. The patient who coughs and has a floating pulse should take principally Hou-pu-ma-huang-tang (Magnolia and Mahuang Combination).

5 liang magnolia bark

4 liang mahuang

2 liang dried ginger

2 liang asarum

gypsum (the size of an egg)

0.5 sheng apricot seed

0.5 sheng pinellia

1 sheng wheat

0.5 sheng schizandra

Cook the wheat in 12 sheng of water until it is well done. Discard the dregs, add the other herbs and decoct the mixture until 3 sheng remains. One sheng warmed is taken three times daily.

第九节　咳而脉沉者,泽漆汤主之。

泽漆汤方:半夏半升,紫参五两(一作紫苑),泽漆三斤(以东流水五斗,煮取一斗五升),生姜五两,白前五两,甘草、黄芩、人参、桂枝各三两。

上九味,㕮咀,内泽漆汁中,煮取五升,温服五合,至夜尽。

9. A patient who coughs and has a submerged pulse should be treated principally with Ze-qi-tang (Helioscopia Combination).

0.5 sheng pinellia

5 liang zi sheng (or aster)

5 liang flesh ginger

5 liang cynanchum

3 liang licorice

3 liang scute

3 liang ginseng

3 liang cinnamon

48 liang helioscopia decocted with 50 sheng of water which flowed eastward until 15 sheng remains

Shred the first eight ingredients and then add to the helioscopia decoction. Decoct the solution again until 5 sheng remains. 0.5 sheng warmed is taken at a time. The entire mixture must be consumed before nightfall.

第十节　火逆上气,咽喉不利,止逆下气,麦门冬汤主之。

麦门冬汤方:麦门冬七升,半夏一升,人参三两,甘草二两,粳米三合,大枣十二枚。

上六味,以水一斗二升,煮取六升,温服一升,日三夜一服。

10. The patient with an adverse cough, flushing of Qi and throat discomfort should be treated principally with Mai-men-dong-tang (Ophiopogon Combination) in order to suppress the adversity and make Qi descend.

7 sheng ophiopogon

1 sheng pinellia

3 ge non-glutinous rice

3 liang ginseng

2 liang licorice

12 pcs. jujube fruits

Decoct the ingredients in 12 sheng of water until 6 sheng remains. One sheng warmed is taken three times during the day and once at night.

第十一节　肺痈喘不得卧,葶苈大枣泻肺汤主之。

葶苈大枣泻肺汤方:葶苈(熬令黄色,捣丸为弹子大),大枣十二枚。

上先以水三升,煮枣取二升,去枣,内葶苈,煮取一升,顿服。

11. A patient with a pulmonary abscess who coughs so severely that he cannot lie down should be treated principally with Ting-li-da-zao-xie-fei-tang (Lepidium and Jujube Combination).

lepidium (simmered until yellow and pounded　　12 jujube traits

into pieces the size of a bullet)

First decoct the jujube in 3 sheng of water until 2 sheng remains, then discard the jujube and add lepidium. Decoct the solution again until 1 sheng remains. The decoction is taken all in one draft.

第十二节　咳而胸满,振寒脉数,咽干不渴,时出浊唾腥臭,久久吐脓如米粥者,为肺痈,桔梗汤主之。

桔梗汤方:桔梗一两,甘草二两。

上二味,以水三升,煮取一升,分温再服,则吐脓血也。

12. Symptoms such as cough with chest distention, shivering, a quick pulse, dry throat, absence of thirst, and frequent expectoration of thick and fishy sputum, eventually expectoration of pus like rice congee (as the disease persists), are evidences of pulmonary abscess. A pulmonary abscess principally requires Jie-geng-tang (Platycodon Combination).

1 liang platycodon　　　　　　　　　　2 liang raw licorice

Decoct the two ingredients in 3 sheng of water until 1 sheng remains. After discarding the dregs the decoction is divided into two portions and one portion is taken warmed twice a day. Thereafter, the patient will emit purulent blood.

第十三节　咳而上气,此为肺胀,其人喘,目如脱状,脉浮大者,越婢加半夏汤主之。

越婢加半夏汤方:麻黄六两,石膏半斤,生姜三两,大枣十五枚,甘草二两,半夏半升。

上六味,以水六升,先煎麻黄,去上沫,内诸药,煮取三升,分温三服。

13. A cough with flushing of Qi due to pulmonary distention that causes asthma and makes the eyes protrude will also produce a floating and big pulse. The afflicted should be principally treated with Yue-pi-jia-ban-xia-tang (Mahuang, Gypsum, and Pinellia Combination).

6 liang mahuang　　　　　　　　　　12 pcs. jujube fruits

8 liang gypsum　　　　　　　　　　　2 liang licorice

3 liang fresh ginger　　　　　　　　　0.5 sheng pinellia

Decoct the mahuang in 6 sheng of water, skim off the foam, add the other ingredients, and decoct until 3 sheng remains. Discard the dregs and take the decoction warmed in three equal doses.

第十四节　肺胀咳而上气,烦躁而喘,脉浮者,心下有水,小青龙加石膏汤主之。

小青龙加石膏汤方:麻黄、芍药、桂枝、细辛、甘草、干姜各三两,五味子、半夏各半升,石膏二两。

上九味,以水一斗,先煮麻黄,去上沫,内诸药,煮取三升。强人服一升,羸者减之,日三服。小儿服四合。

14. Pulmonary distention with cough and flushing up of Qi, annoyance and irritation along with asthma, and a floating pulse portends water stagnated beneath the heart; the conformation principally needs Xiao-qing-long-jia-shi-gao-tang(Minor Blue Dragon and Gypsum Combination).

3 liang mahuang	3 liang licorice
3 liang cinnamon	2 liang gypsum
3 liang peony	0.5 sheng schizandra
3 liang asarum	0.5 sheng pinellia
3 liang dried ginger	

Decoct the mahuang in 10 sheng of water, skim off the floating foam, then add the other ingredients and decoct until three sheng remains. Discard the dregs and take the decoction warmed according to regimen: strong patients take one sheng of the decoction three times daily; children take 0.4 sheng; and weak patients less than one sheng.

Six other formulas treat lung atrophy or lung abscess.

炙甘草汤,治肺痿涎唾多,心中温温液液者。

Zhi-gan-cao-tang(Baked Licorice Combination) treats pulmonary asthenia, excessive saliva and drivel, agitatation and discomfort in the heart.

甘草汤:甘草二两。
上一味,以水三升,煮减半,分温三服。

Gan-cao-tang(Licorice Decoction) treats the same symptoms as Baked Licorice Combination except it also helps stop hemorrhaging.

2 liang licorice

Decoct the licorice with 3 sheng of water until it reduces by half. Drain to discard the dregs and take the decoction warmed in three equal doses.

生姜甘草汤：治肺痿咳唾涎沫不止，咽燥而渴。

生姜五两，人参三两，甘草四两，大枣十五枚。

上四味，以水七升，煮取三升，分温三服。

Sheng-jiang-gan-cao-tang（Fresh Ginger and Licorice Combination）treats pulmonary asthenia with incessant coughing and expectoration of saliva and drivel, pharyngeal dryness, and thirst.

5 liang fresh ginger	3 liang ginseng
4 liang licorice	15 pcs. jujube fruits

Decoct the ingredients in 7 sheng of water until 3 sheng remains. Discard the dregs and take the decoction warmed in three equal doses.

桂枝去芍药加皂荚汤：治肺痿吐涎沫。

桂枝、生姜各三两，甘草二两，大枣十枚，皂荚一枚（去皮子，炙焦）。

上五味，以水七升，微微火煮，取三升，分温三服。

Gui-zhi-qu-shao-yao-jia-zao-jia-tang（Cinnamon and Gleditsia Combination）treats pulmonary asthenia with expectoration of drivel and frothy saliva.

3 liang cinnamon	3 liang fresh ginger
2 liang licorice	10 pcs. jujube fruits

1 gleditsia capsule with outer skin and inner seeds removed, then baked to a charred state

Decoct the ingredients in 7 sheng of water over a low fire until 3 sheng remains, discard the dregs, and divide the decoction into three equal portions. Each portion is taken warmed three times a day.

《外台》桔梗白散：治咳而胸满，振寒脉数，咽干不渴，时出浊唾腥臭，久久吐脓如米粥者，为肺痈。

桔梗、贝母各三分。巴豆一分（去皮，熬研如脂）。

上三味，为散，强人饮服半钱匕，羸者减之。病在膈上者吐脓血，膈下者泻出，若下多不止，饮冷水一杯则定。

Jie-geng-bai-san（Platycodon and Croton Formula）is for symptoms such as cough with chest distention, shivering, quick pulse, dry throat, absence of thirst, frequent expectoration of thick and fishy smelling sputum and eventually expectoration of pus like rice congee（as the disease persists）, which reflects pulmonary abscess.

3 fen platycodon	3 fen fritillaria

1 fen croton with seed coat removed and the seed stewed and ground into a cream

Pulverize the ingredients and mix together. Strong patients take one half qianbi of the powder;

weak patients require a reduced dose. If the disease is located above the diaphragm, the patient will expectorate pus. If the disease is located below the diaphragm, he will have diarrhea. If diarrhea occurs incessantly, one cup of cold water will stop it.

《千金》苇茎汤：治咳有微热，烦满，胸中甲错，是为肺痈。

苇茎二升，薏苡仁半升，桃仁五十枚，瓜瓣半升。

上四味，以水一斗，先煮苇茎，得五升，去滓，内诸药，煮取二升，服一升，再服，当吐如脓。

Wei-jing-tang (Phragmites Stem Combination) helps a cough with mild fever, annoying distention, and coarse and scaly skin on the chest-symptoms of pulmonary abscess.

2 sheng phragmites stems	50 persica seeds
0.5 sheng coix	0.5 sheng benincasa seeds

Decoct phragmites stems in 10 sheng of water until 5 sheng remains, discard the dregs, add the other ingredients, decoct again until 2 sheng remains. Take one sheng followed by another. The patient will expectorate purulent matter.

第十五节　肺痈，胸满胀，一身面目浮肿，鼻塞，清涕出，不闻香臭酸辛，咳逆上气，喘鸣迫塞，葶苈大枣泻肺汤主之。（方见上，三日一剂，可至三四剂，此先服小青龙汤一剂乃进，小青龙汤方见咳嗽门中）

15. Pulmonary abscess exhibiting chest fullness and distention; generalized edema; a stuffy, runny nose and loss of smell; adverse cough with flushing up of Qi; asthma and stridor; and a compressed feeling in the chest should be principally treated with Ting-li-da-zao-xie-fei-tang (Lepidium and Jujube Combination). One sheng is taken warmed every three days; a total of three to four sheng of the formula may be taken. Before taking this formula, each time one dose of Xiao-qing-long-tang (Minor Blue Dragon Combination) should be taken.

奔豚气病脉证治第八

VIII.
On pulse Syndrome Complex and Treatment of
the Qi Disease Ben Tun

第一节　师曰:病有奔豚,有吐脓,有惊怖,有火邪,此四部病,皆从惊发得之。

1. The master said: "Fright causes four conditions – Ben tun, expectoration of pus, panic, and fire evil."

第二节　师曰:奔豚病从少腹起,上冲咽喉,发作欲死,复还止,皆从惊恐得之。

2. The master said: "Ben tun syndrome originates in the lower abdomen and rushes upward to the throat. An attack of the syndrome causes the patient unbearable suffering, which gradually reduces and subsides. The cause of the disease is fright and terror."

第三节　奔豚气上冲胸,腹痛,往来寒热,奔豚汤主之。
奔豚汤方:甘草、穹劳、当归各二两,半夏四两,黄芩二两,生葛五两,芍药二两,生姜四两,甘李根白皮一升。
上九味,以水二斗,煮取五升,温服一升,日三服,夜一服。

3. Ben tun with Qi rushing toward the chest, abdominal aching, and alternating chills and fever essentially requires treatment with Ben-tun-tang (Pueraria and Ginger Combination).

2 liang licorice	5 liang fresh pueraria
2 liang cnidium	2 liang peony
2 liang tang-kuei	4 liang fresh ginger
4 liang pinellia	1 sheng white bark from the root of communis
2 liang scute	

Decoct the ingredients in 20 sheng of water until 5 sheng remains. One sheng warmed is taken three times during the day and once at night.

第四节　发汗后,烧针令其汗,针处被寒,核起而赤者,必发奔豚,气从小腹上至心,灸其核上各一壮,与桂枝加桂汤主之。

桂枝加桂汤方:桂枝五两,芍药三两,甘草二两(炙),生姜三两,大枣十二枚。

上五味,以水七升,微火煮取三升,去滓,温服一升。

4. If acupuncture with a burning needle is applied following a sweating treatment and a swelling red nucleus develops on the site of needle insertion as a consequence of chill-evil invasion at the site, Ben tun will definitely ensue with Qi rushing from the lower abdomen toward the heart. The treatment of this condition calls for the application of one unit of moxibustion on each nucleus and the administration of Gui-zhi-jia-gui-tang (Cinnamon, Licorice, and Ginger Combination).

5 liang cinnamon	3 liang fresh ginger
3 liang peony	12 pcs. jujube fruits
2 liang baked licorice	

Decoct the ingredients in 7 sheng of water on a low fire until 3 sheng remains; discard the dregs. One sheng warmed is taken.

第五节　发汗后脐下悸者,欲作奔豚,茯苓桂枝甘草大枣汤主之。

茯苓桂枝甘草大枣汤方:茯苓半斤,甘草二两(炙),大枣十五枚,桂枝四两。

上四味,以甘澜水一斗,先煮茯苓,减二升,内诸药,煮取三升,去滓,温服一升,日三服。

5. Palpitation beneath the umbilicus following a sweating treatment portends a Ben tun seizure. Fu-ling-gui-zhi-gan-cao-da-zao-tang (Hoelen, Licorice, and Jujube Combination) should be prescribed.

8 liang hoelen	15 pcs. jujube fruits
2 liang baked licorice	4 liang cinnamon

Decoct the hoelen in 10 sheng of aerated water until the volume reduces by 2 sheng; then add the other ingredients and decoct until 3 sheng remains. Discard the dregs. One sheng warmed is taken three times a day.

胸痹心痛短气病脉证治第九

IX.

On Pulse Syndrome Complex and Treatment of Thoracic Paralysis, Heart Pain and Gasping (Shortness of Breath)

第一节 师曰：夫脉当取太过不及，阳微阴弦，即胸痹而痛，所以然者，责其极虚也，今阳虚知在上焦，所以胸痹、心痛者，以其阴弦故也。

1. The master said: "When feeling the pulse, excessiveness and deficiency should be diagnosed. Feebleness at Yang and tightness at Yin indicate a Chest Obstruction syndrome with pain. The extremely deficient state is the causa morbi. Feeble pulse at Yang indicates prevalence of a deficient state at the Upper Portion of Body Cavity. Chest Obstruction and Heart Pain is manifested by a tight pulse at Yin."

第二节 平人无寒热，短气不足以息者，实也。

2. A normal person who is not suffering from either a fever or a chill may feel a shortness of breath with hypopnea. This is an excessive case.

第三节 胸痹之病，喘息咳唾，胸背痛，短气，寸口脉沉而迟，关上小紧数，栝蒌薤白白酒汤主之。

栝蒌薤白白酒汤方：栝蒌实一枚(捣)，薤白半升，白酒七升。

上三味，同煮，取二升，分温再服。

3. Chest Obstruction syndrome has the symptoms and signs of panting, coughing, spitting, shortness of breath and pain in the chest and back. The pulse is deep and slow in the Inch and slender-tense-speedy in the Bar should be treated principally with Gua-lou-xie-bai-bai-jiu-tang (Trichosanthes, Bakeri, and Vinegar Combination).

7 sheng vinegar   the seed from 1 pc. trichosanthes fruit pounded

0.5 sheng bakeri

Decoct the three ingredients together until 2 sheng remains. The solution is divided into two portions. One portion is taken warmed twice daily.

第四节　胸痹不得卧，心痛彻背者，栝蒌薤白半夏汤主之。

栝蒌薤白半夏汤方：栝蒌实一枚（捣），薤白三两，半夏半斤，白酒一斗。

上四味，同煮，取四升，温服一升，日三服。

4. Chest obstruction syndrome so painful that the patient can not lie flat principally because of dragging pain that penetrates the back should be treated with Gua-lou-xie-bai-ban-xia-tang (Trichosanthes, Bakeri, and Pinellia Combination).

| the seed from 1 pc. trichosanthes fruit pounded | 8 liang pinellia |
| 3 liang bakeri | 10 sheng vinegar |

Decoct the four ingredients together until 4 sheng remains. One sheng warmed is taken three times a day.

第五节　胸痹心中痞气，留气结在胸，胸满，胁下逆抢心，枳实薤白桂枝汤主之；人参汤亦主之。

枳实薤白桂枝汤方：枳实四枚，厚朴四两，薤白半斤，桂枝一两，栝蒌实一枚（捣）。

上五味，以水五升，先煮枳实、厚朴，取二升，去滓，内诸药，煮数沸，分温三服。

人参汤方：人参、甘草、干姜、白术各三两。

上四味，以水八升，煮取三升，温服一升，日三服。

5. Chest obstruction syndrome accompanied either by obstructed Qi beneath the heart or by bound Qi with distention in the chest and ribs and flushing Qi from the hypochondria to the heart should be treated with either Ren-sheng-tang (Ginseng and Ginger Combination) or Zhi-shi-xie-bai-gui-zhi-tang (Zhi-shi, Bakeri, and Cinnamon Combination).

4 pcs. Zhi-shi fruits	8 liang bakeri
4 liang magnolia bark	the seed from 1 pc. trichosanthes fruit pounded
1 liang cinnamon	

Decoct the first two ingredients in 5 sheng of water until 2 sheng remains. Discard the dregs, add the remaining herbs, and boil for a while. The decoction is divided into three portions and taken warmed three times a day.

Ginseng and Ginger Combination

| 3 liang ginseng | 3 liang dried ginger |
| 3 liang licorice | 3 liang atractylodes |

Decoct the ingredients with 8 sheng of water until 3 sheng remains. One sheng warmed is taken three times a day (Zhi-shi, Bakeri, and Cinnamon Combination).

第六节　胸痹,胸中气塞,短气,茯苓杏仁甘草汤主之;橘枳姜汤亦主之。
茯苓杏仁甘草汤方:茯苓三两,杏仁五十个,甘草一两。
上三味,以水一斗,煮取五升,温服一升,日三服。不差,更服。
橘枳姜汤方:橘皮一斤,枳实三两,生姜半斤。
上三味,以水五升,煮取二升,分温再服。

6. Chest obstruction syndrome should be principally treated with Ju-zhi-jiang-tang (Auran-tium, Zhi-shi, and Ginger Combination) if the main symptom is Qi obstruction in the chest or with Fu-ling-xing-ren-gan-cao-tang (Hoelen, Apricot Seed, and Licorice Combination) if the main symptom is shortness of breath.

Aurantium, zhi-shi, and Ginger Combination:

16 liang aurantium　　　　　　　　　　8 liang fresh ginger

3 liang zhi-shi

Decoct the ingredients in 5 sheng of water until 2 sheng remains. Divide into two portions. Each is taken warmed.

Hoelen, Apricot, and Licorice Combination

3 liang hoelen　　　　　　　　　　50 pcs. apricot seeds

1 liang licorice

Decoct the ingredients in 10 sheng of water until 5 sheng remains. One sheng warmed is taken three times daily. A second dose is required if the first dose is not effective.

第七节　胸痹缓急者,薏苡附子散主之。
薏苡附子散方:薏苡仁十五两,大附子十枚(炮)。
上二味,杵为散,服方寸匕,日三服。

7. Chest obstruction syndrome which aches mildly with occasional episodes of severe aching should be treated with Yi-yi-fu-zhi-san (Coix and Aconite Formula).

15 liang coix　　　　　　　　　　10 pcs. large baked aconites

Pound the ingredients into powder. One fangcunbi of the powder is taken three times daily.

第八节　心中痞,诸逆心悬痛,桂枝生姜枳实汤主之。
桂枝生姜枳实汤方:桂枝、生姜各三两,枳实五枚。
上三味,以水六升,煮取三升,分温三服。

8. Chest obstruction syndrome with hypochondrial adverse flushing causing heart pain should

be treated with Gui-zhi-sheng-jiang-zhi-shi-tang (Cinnamon, Ginger, and Zhi-shi Combination).

3 liang cinnamon   5 pcs. zhi-shi fruits

3 liang fresh ginger

Decoct the ingredients in 6 sheng of water until 3 sheng remains. Divide into three portions. A portion is taken warmed three times daily.

第九节　心痛彻背，背痛彻心，乌头赤石脂丸主之。

乌头赤石脂丸方：蜀椒一两(一法二分)，乌头一分(炮)，附子半两(炮)(一法一分)，干姜一两(一法一分)，赤石脂一两(一法二分)。

上五味，末之，蜜丸如梧桐子大，先食服一丸，日三服。不知，稍加服。

9. Heart Pain with dragging pain leading towards the back and back pain with dragging pain leading to the cardia can be treated with Wu-tou-chi-shi-zhi-wan (Wu-tou and Kaolin Formula).

1 liang zanthoxylum   1 fen baked wu-tou

1 liang dried ginger   50 fen baked aconite

1 liang kaolin (red bole)

Pulverize the ingredients, knead with honey, and make into pills as large as a sterculia seed. One pill is taken before each meal. If no effect occurs, the dosage should be slightly increased.

九痛丸：治九种心痛。

附子三两(炮)，生狼牙一两(炙香)，巴豆一两(去皮心，熬，研如脂)，人参、干姜、吴茱萸各一两。

上六味，末之，炼蜜丸如桐子大，酒下。强人初服三丸，日三服；弱者二丸。兼治卒中恶，腹胀痛，口不能言；又治连年积冷，流注心胸痛，并冷冲上气，落马坠车血疾等，皆主之。忌口如常法。

Jiu-tong-wan (Aconite and Croton Formula) treats nine kinds of heart pain. This formula also treats sudden fainting or acute contractions of vicious Qi resulting in abdominal distention and aching, and aphrasia; chronic chills that flow about and cause aching of the heart and chest and flushing up of chill Qi; injuries from falls from a horse or from a cart; and blood diseases. Ordinary eating taboos to drug administration apply to this formula.

3 liang baked aconite   1 liang flesh potentilla, baked until fragrant

1 liang ginseng   1 liang croton seeds with seed coat and core

1 liang evodia   removed, stewed and ground into a cream

1 liang dried ginger

Pulverize the ingredients, knead with honey, and make into pills the size of a sterculia seed. Three pills for strong patients, or two pills for weak patients, are taken with wine three times daily.

腹满寒疝宿食病脉证治第十

X.

On Pulse Syndrome Complex and Treatment of Abdominal Distention, Chill Colic and Over Undigested Food

第一节　趺阳脉微弦,法当腹满,不满者必便难,两胠疼痛,此虚寒从下上也,当以温药服之。

1. Feeble and tight Fuyang pulse generally indicates abdominal distention. If there is no abdominal distention, there will be constipation, pain on costal regions caused by the ascending of Deficiency and Cold. A warming agent should be served.

第二节　病者腹满,按之不痛为虚,痛者为实,可下之。舌黄未下者,下之黄自去。

2. A distended abdomen that does not ache when pressed is due to weakness; if the abdomen aches, there is firmness and purging is needed. The yellow color on the tongue will disappear after purgation.

第三节　腹满时减,复如故,此为寒,当与温药。

3. Abdominal distention which leaves at times but resumes after is due to chills and should be treated with warm drugs.

第四节　病者痿黄,燥而不渴,胸中寒实而利不止者,死。

4. A patient with a withered, yellowish complexion, agitation but no thirst, a firm chill in the chest, and incessant diarrhea is incurable.

第五节　寸口脉弦者,即胁下拘急而痛,其人啬啬恶寒也。

5. Pulse at the Inch (under the first finger) is tight. The patient has chills, contractions and pain throughout the costal regions.

第六节　夫中寒家,喜欠。其人清涕出,发热色和者,善嚏。

6. A patient with internal chills frequently yawns. If he has a runny nose with a fever and a normal complexion, he will sneeze readily.

第七节　中寒,其人下利,以里虚也,欲嚏不能,此人肚中寒。

7. A patient with internal chills has diarrhea because the interior is weak; if he wants to sneeze but can not, it is because he has chills (or pain) in his stomach.

第八节　夫瘦人绕脐痛,必有风冷,谷气不行,而反下之,其气必冲,不冲者,心下则痞。

8. A thin individual with pain around the navel and an accumulation of undigested food must have contracted wind cold. A purgative, instead of a warm drug, will flush Qi. If Qi does not flush, obstruction beneath the heart will develop.

第九节　病腹满,发热十日,脉浮而数,饮食如故,厚朴七物汤主之。
厚朴七物汤方:厚朴半斤,甘草、大黄各三两,大枣十枚,枳实五枚,桂枝二两,生姜五两。
上七味,以水一斗,煮取四升,温服八合,日三服。呕者加半夏五合,下利去大黄,寒多者加生姜至半斤。

9. A person suffering from abdominal distention with fever for ten days who has a floating and quick pulse and eats and drinks as usual should take Hou-pu-qi-wu-tang (Magnolia Seven Combination).

8 liang magnolia bark	10 pcs. jujubes
3 liang licorice	5 pcs. zhi-shi fruits
3 liang rhubarb	5 liang fresh ginger
2 liang cinnamon	

Decoct the ingredients in 10 sheng of water until 4 sheng remains. Eight ge warmed is taken three times daily. For vomiting, add 0.5 sheng of pinellia; for diarrhea, delete rhubarb; for chills, increase the fresh ginger to 0.5 jin.

第十节　腹中寒气,雷鸣切痛,胸胁逆满,呕吐,附子粳米汤主之。

附子粳米汤方:附子一枚(炮),半夏、粳米各半升,甘草一两,大枣十枚。

上五味,以水八升,煮米熟,汤成,去滓,温服一升,日三服。

10. Fu-zi-jing-mi-tang (Aconite and Oryza Combination) treats chills in the abdomen with borborygmus and severe aching, adverse chest and rib distention, and vomiting.

1 pc. baked aconite	10 pcs. jujube fruits
0.5 sheng pinellia	0.5 sheng non-glutinous rice
1 liang licorice	

Decoct the ingredients in 8 sheng of water until the rice is well done, then discard the dregs and take one sheng of the decoction warmed three times daily.

第十一节　痛而闭者,厚朴三物汤主之。

厚朴三物汤方:厚朴八两,大黄四两,枳实五枚。

上三味,以水一斗二升,先煮二味,取五升,内大黄,煮取三升,温服一升。以利为度。

11. Hou-pu-san-wu-tang (Magnolia Three Combination) treats aching with obstructive conditions, such as stomach distention or constipation.

8 liang magnolia bark　　　　5 pcs. zhi-shi fruits

4 liang rhubarb

Decoct the ingredients except rhubarb in 12 sheng of water until 5 sheng remains; then add rhubarb and decoct again until 3 sheng remains. Take one sheng warmed consecutively until a bowel movement occurs.

第十二节　按之心下满痛者,此为实也,当下之,宜大柴胡汤。

大柴胡汤方:柴胡半斤,黄芩三两,芍药三两,半夏半升(洗),枳实四枚(炙),大黄二两,大枣十二枚,生姜五两。

上八味,以水一斗二升,煮取六升,去滓,温服一升,日三服。

12. Distention and aching beneath the heart due to firm evil should be purged with Da-chai-hu-tang (Major Bupleurum Combination) as the preferred drug.

8 liang bupleurum	0.5 sheng washed pinellia
3 liang scute	4 pcs. baked zhi-shi fruits
3 liang peony	12 pcs. jujube fruits
2 liang rhubarb	5 liang fresh ginger

Decoct the ingredients in 12 sheng of water until 6 sheng remains. Discard the dregs and decoct again until 3 sheng remains. One sheng warmed is taken three times daily.

第十三节 腹满不减,减不足言,当须下之,宜大承气汤。大承气汤方:见前痉病中。

13. Abdominal distention which remains unreduced or only slightly reduced should be purged with Da-cheng-qi-tang (Major Rhubarb Combination) as the preferred drug.

第十四节 心胸中大寒痛,呕不能饮食,腹中寒,上冲皮起出见有头足,上下痛而不可触近,大建中汤主之。

大建中汤方:蜀椒二合(炒去汗),干姜四两,人参二两。

上三味,以水四升,煮取二升,去滓,内胶饴一升,微火煎取一升半,分温再服;如一炊顷,可饮粥二升,后更服。当一日食糜,温覆之。

14. A patient with strong chilling pain in the heart and chest, vomiting that prevents eating, chills in the abdomen and bulging of the abdominal skin due to flushing of chills, and skin so painful on both surface and underside as to be untouchable needs Da-jian-zhong-tang (Major Zanthoxylum Combination).

2 ge zanthoxylum fried to expel the oil   4 liang dried ginger

2 liang ginseng

Decoct the herbs in 4 sheng of water until 2 sheng remains. Discard the dregs and add 1 sheng of maltose. Decoct on a mild fire until 1.5 sheng remains. Divide into two portions. One portion is taken warmed. After a period about the same as one spends in cooking a meal (about 30 minutes) has elapsed, 2 sheng of hot rice congee followed by the second portion of the drug warmed should be drunk. On that day the patient should eat rice glue (thicker than congee) all day long and cover himself with quilts to keep warm.

第十五节 胁下偏痛,发热,其脉紧弦,此寒也,以温药下之,宜大黄附子汤。

大黄附子汤方:大黄三两,附子二枚(炮),细辛二两。

上三味,以水五升,煮取二升,分温三服;若强人煮取二升半,分温三服。服后如人行四、五里,进一服。

15. Unilateral pain beneath the ribs, fever, and a tense and chordal pulse portend chills. The condition calls for purging with warm drugs such as Da-huang-fu-zi-tang (Rhubarb and Aconite Combination).

3 liang rhubarb   3 pcs. baked aconite roots

2 liang asarum

Decoct the ingredients in 5 sheng of water until 2 sheng remains and divide into three portions.

One portion warmed is taken three times daily. For strong patients decoct until 2.5 sheng remains and divide into three portions. One portion is taken warmed three times daily. A specific regimen for this drug is one portion is taken after which another portion is taken at intervals as long as it takes to walk 4 to 5 Li.

第十六节　寒气厥逆,赤丸主之。

赤丸方:茯苓四两,半夏四两(洗),乌头二两(炮),细辛一两。

上四味,末之,内真朱为色,炼蜜丸如麻子大,先食酒饮下三丸,日再夜一服;不知,稍增之,以知为度。

16. Chill Qi causing cold extremities requires Chi-wan(Wu-tou and Pinellia Formula).

4 liang hoelen	2 liang baked wu-tou
4 liang washed pinellia	1 liang asarum

Grind the four ingredients to powder, add cinnabar as acolorant, and knead the mixture with honey. Make the mass into pills the size of a cannabis seed. Three pills are taken with wine before meals two times a day and once at night. If no effect is observed, the dose is increased a little at a time until effective.

第十七节　腹痛,脉弦而紧,弦则卫气不行,即恶寒,紧则不欲食,邪正相搏,则为寒疝。寒疝绕脐痛,若发则白汗出,手足厥冷,其脉沉紧("沉紧",一作"沉弦")者,大乌头煎主之。

大乌头煎方:乌头大者五枚(熬,去皮,不㕮咀)。

上以水三升,煮取一升,去滓,内蜜二升,煎令水气尽,取二升,强人服七合,弱人服五合。不差,明日更服,不可一日再服。

17. Abdominal aching and a chordal and tense pulse represent a condition known as chillphobia; the chordal characteristic indicates stagnancy of the surface protective Qi and the tension, anorexia. Conflict between normal Qi and evil Qi gives rise to chill colic. A seizure of chill colic generates aching around the navel, spontaneous sweating, cold arms and legs, and a submerged and tense pulse. Both conditions call for Da-wu-tou-jian (Wu-tou and Honey Combination).

5 pcs. large wu tou simmered to honey remove the skin (do not shred)

Decoct the wu tou in 3 sheng of water until one sheng remains, discard the dregs, add 2 sheng of honey, and decoct until all the water content has evaporated off and 2 sheng remains. Strong patients take 7 ge, weak patients 5 ge. If no effect is shown, another dose is taken the next day. The patient should never take two doses in one day.

第十八节　寒疝,腹中痛及胁痛里急者,当归生姜羊肉汤主之。

当归生姜羊肉汤方：当归三两,生姜五两,羊肉一斤。

上三味,以水八升,煮取三升,温服七合,日三服。若寒多者加生姜成一斤;痛多而呕者加橘皮二两,白术一两。加生姜者亦加水五升,煮取三升二合,服之。

18. Chill colic with abdominal aching, pain in the ribs, and an urgent internal feeling requires Dang-gui-sheng-jiang-yang-rou-tang (Dang-gui, Ginger, and Mutton Combination).

3 liang dang-gui   16 liang mutton

5 liang fresh ginger

Decoct the three ingredients in 8 sheng of water until 3 sheng remains. Seven ge warmed is taken three times daily. If the patient experiences more chills, increase the amount of fresh ginger up to one catty; if the patient has more aching with vomiting, add 2 liang of citrus peel and 1 liang of atractylodes. With the increase in fresh ginger, add an additional 5 sheng of water and decoct until 3.2 sheng remains.

第十九节　寒疝腹中痛,逆冷,手足不仁,若身疼痛,灸,刺,诸药不能治,抵当乌头桂枝汤主之。

乌头桂枝汤方：乌头。

上一味,以蜜二斤,煎减半,去滓,以桂枝汤五合解之,得一升后,初服二合;不知,即服三合;又不知,复加至五合。其知者,如醉状,得吐者为中病。

桂枝汤方：桂枝三两(去皮),芍药三两,甘草二两(炙),生姜三两,大枣十二枚。

上五味,剉,以水七升微火煮取三升,去滓。

19. Chill colic with abdominal aching, adverse chills, cold and numb extremities, and generalized aching unresponsive to moxibustion, acupuncture, and other drugs should be treated with Wu-tou-gui-zhi-tang (Wu-tou and Cinnamon Combination).

wu tou

Decoct wu tou in 2 jin of honey until the decoction is reduced by half. Discard the dregs and mix the wu tou decoction with 5 ge of Gui-zhi-tang (Cinnamon Combination, prepared as indicated below) and boil until the volume is reduced to 1 sheng. 2 ge is taken at the beginning. If no effect occurs, the dosage is increased to 3 ge. If again no effect is shown, it is increased to 5 ge. A drunken appearance in the patient and vomiting imply the drug has taken effect.

3 liang decorticated cinnamon   3 liang fresh ginger

3 liang peony   12 pcs. jujubes

2 liang baked licorice

Shred the ingredients and decoct with 7 sheng of water on a mild fire until 3 sheng remains. Discard the dregs.

第二十节 其脉数而紧,乃弦,状如弓弦,按之不移;脉数弦者,当下其寒;脉紧大而迟者,必心下坚;脉大而紧者,阳中有阴,可下之。

20. A chordal pulse resembles a vibrating bow string – quick and tense. Also it feels stationary. A chordal and quick pulse calls for purgation to discharge the chill. The patient with a tense, big, and slow pulse will have hardening beneath the heart, or if the pulse is tense and big only, either condition denoting the presence of yin within yang, he or she also needs purgation.

[Other applicable formulas follow]

《外台》乌头汤:治寒疝腹中绞痛,贼风入攻五脏,拘急不得转侧,发作有时,使人阴缩,手足厥逆。

Wu-tou-tang (Wu-tou Combination) treats chill colic in the abdomen, visceral spasms preventing turning of the body as a consequence of evil-wind intrusion. Seizures occur at definite times, causing scrotal retraction and chilling of the limbs.

《外台》柴胡桂枝汤方:治心腹卒中痛者。柴胡四两,黄芩、人参、芍药、桂枝、生姜各一两半,甘草一两,半夏二合半,大枣六枚。
上九味,以水六升,煮取三升,温服一升,日三服。

Chai-hu-gui-zhi-tang (Bupleurum and Cinnamon Combination) treats acute pain of the heart and the abdomen.

4.0 liang bupleurum	1.5 liang fresh ginger
1.5 liang scute	1 liang licorice
1.5 liang ginseng	0.25 sheng pinellia
1.5 liang peony	6 pcs. jujube fruits
1.5 liang cinnamon	

Decoct the ingredients in 6 sheng of water until 3 sheng remains. One sheng warmed is taken three times a day.

《外台》走马汤:治中恶心痛腹胀,大便不通。巴豆二枚(去皮心,熬),杏仁二枚。
上二味,以绵缠捶令碎,热汤二合,捻取白汁,饮之,当下。老小量之,通治飞尸鬼击病。

Zou-ma-tang (Croton and Apricot Seed Combination) treats infectious tuberculosis, "ghost attack" (a sudden seizure as if one were stabbed by a knife or beaten with a stick) with symptoms of severe pain in the chest so painful as to be untouchable, and sometimes hematemesis, nosebleeds, or anuria. It also alleviates acute contraction of vicious evil, heart pain, abdominal distention, and constipation.

1 pc. croton seed with seed coat and core removed, stewed

2 pcs. apricot seeds

Wrap the seeds in a piece of linen, then smash them with a hammer. Kneading and squeezing the wrapped package in 2 sheng of hot water produces white juice which is then drunk. It purges. For old and young, dosage is adjusted accordingly.

第二十一节　问曰：人病有宿食，何以别之？师曰：寸口脉浮而大，按之反涩，尺中亦微而涩，故知有宿食，大承气汤主之。

21. The disciples asked: "How can we be sure the patient has yesterday's undigested food within himself?"

The master replied: "Pulse at the Inch (under the first finger) is floating-huge. When it is pressed deeply, it becomes hesitant. Pulse in the Cubit (under the ring-finger) is also feeble-hesitant. This is evidence of indigestion. Decoction of Da-cheng-qi-tang (Major Rhubarb Combination) can be adopted as a purgative."

第二十二节　脉数而滑者，实也，此有宿食，下之愈，宜大承气汤。

22. A quick and slippery pulse reflects fullness (or firmness) from the presence of overnight undigested food. It can be cured by purging principally with Da-cheng-qi-tang (Major Rhubarb Combination).

第二十三节　下利不欲食者，有宿食也，当下之，宜大承气汤。

23. Diarrhea without an appetite is due to food undigested overnight which requires purging with Da-cheng-qi-tang (Major Rhubarb Combination).

第二十四节　宿食在上脘，当吐之，宜瓜蒂散。瓜蒂散方：瓜蒂一分(熬黄)，赤小豆一分(煮)。

上二味，杵为散，以香豉七合煮取汁，和散一钱匕，温服之，不吐者，少加之，以快吐为度而止。亡血及虚者不可与之。

24. Overnight undigested food lodged in the upper stomach should be treated with emetics. Gua-di-san (Melon Peduncle Formula) is suitable for this purpose.

1 fen peduncle simmered　　　　　　　1 fen cooked phaseolus until yellow

Pound the two ingredients into powder, one qianbi of which is taken together with the warmed juice decocted from 0.7 sheng of soya bean relish. Dosage should gradually be increased until the patient vomits readily. It should not be given to patients with loss of blood and weakness conformation.

第二十五节　脉紧如转索无常者，有宿食也。

25 A rope-like pulse alternately tense and slippery indicates the presence of overnight undigested food.

第二十六节　脉紧，头痛风寒，腹中有宿食不化也。

26. A tense pulse with headache signifies wind and chill evils, or the presence of overnight undigested food.

五脏风寒积聚病脉证并治第十一

XI.

On Pulse Syndrome Complex and Treatment of Visceral Wind, Chills, and Tumors

第一节　肺中风者，口燥而喘，身运而重，冒而肿胀。

1. Pulmonary windstroke manifests itself in a dry mouth, asthma, vertigo, generalized heaviness, dizziness, and swelling.

第二节　肺中寒，吐浊涕。

2. With pulmonary chillstroke the afflicted expectorate thick sputum.

第三节　肺死脏，浮之虚，按之弱如葱叶，下无根者死。

3. The appearance of a genuine pulmonary pulse-empty on light palpation and weak and bottomless as a scallion leaf on heavy palpation-signals impending death.

第四节　肝中风者，头目瞤，两胁痛，行常伛，令人嗜甘。

4. The patient with liver windstroke exhibits trembling of the head and eyes, bilateral rib pain, a hunched posture when walking, and a fondness for sweets.

第五节　肝中寒者，两臂不举，舌本燥，喜太息，胸中痛，不得转侧，食则吐而汗出也。

5. Liver chillstroke induces an inability to raise either arm, a dry tongue, frequent sighing, an aching chest making it impossible to turn over, and vomiting with sweating after eating.

第六节　肝死脏,浮之弱,按之如索不来,或曲如蛇行者,死。

6. The presence of the genuine hepatic pulse – weak on light palpation and unresisting as a hanging rope or undulatory like a moving snake on heavy palpation – portends death.

第七节　肝著,其人常欲蹈其胸上,先未苦时,但欲饮热,旋覆花汤主之。
旋覆花汤方：旋覆花三两,葱十四茎,新绛少许。
上三法,以水三升,煮取一升,顿服之。

7. A patient with liver stagnation often feels like he wants someone to tread on his chest. Before becoming afflicted he desires hot drinks. The condition calls primarily for Xuan-fu-hua-tang (Inula Combination).

3 liang inula flowers　　　　　　　　　swatch of new red cloth（dyed with rubia or
14 pcs. stems allium　　　　　　　　　carthamus）
Decoct the three ingredients in 3 sheng of water until one sheng remains. All the decoction is taken in one draft.

第八节　心中风者,翕翕发热,不能起,心中饥,食即呕吐。

8. Cardiac windstroke manifests a thriving fever, an inability to arise, a hungry feeling in the heart, and vomiting following eating.

第九节　心中寒者,其人苦病心如啖蒜状,剧者心痛彻背,背痛彻心,譬如蛊注;其脉浮者,自吐乃愈。

9. A person with chills in the heart experiences a peculiar type of cardiac distress similar to that following the ingestion of garlic; in the most severe cases the pain will radiate to the back from the heart, or vice versa, very much like Gu zhu disease. If the patient's pulse is floating, he may recover after treatment with emesis.

第十节　心伤者,其人劳倦,即头面赤而下重,心中痛而自烦,发热,当脐跳,其脉弦,此为心脏伤所致也。

10. A patient with heart injury exhibits lassitude, reddening of the head and face, heaviness in the lower torso, pain and discomfort in the heart, fever, throbbing at the navel, and achordal pulse.

第十一节　心死脏,浮之实如麻豆,按之益躁急者,死。

11. The presence of a genuine heart pulse – solid as a rolling bean when palpated superficially but more agitated and quick on heavy palpation – protends death.

第十二节　邪哭使魂魄不安者,血气少也;血气少者属于心,心气虚者,其人则畏,合目欲眠,梦远行而精神离散,魂魄妄行。阴气衰者为癫,阳气衰者为狂。

12. Unreasonable crying and accompanying mental uneasiness are due to blood and Qi deficiencies connected to the heart. A patient with cardiac Qi deficiency will always be fearful. The moment he closes his eyes to fall asleep he dreams of going to a distant place, his spirit disintegrating and his soul wandering aimlessly. Deterioration of yin Qi leads to dian (epilepsey) and deterioration of yang Qi to kuang (mania).

第十三节　脾中风者,翕翕发热,形如醉人,腹中烦重,皮目瞤瞤而短气。

13. Thriving fever, a drunkard's appearance, abdominal heaviness with annoyance, and twitching of the skin and eyes together with gasping characterizes splenic windstroke.

第十四节　脾死脏,浮之大坚,按之如覆杯,洁洁状如摇者死。

14. A genuine splenic pulse – on light palpation big and firm and on heavy palpation like an up-side-down cup (hollow and empty inside and with no liquid dripping) – unstably swings to and fro with occasional abrupt interruptions. It predicts death.

第十五节　趺阳脉浮而涩,浮则胃气强,涩则小便数,浮涩相抟,大便则坚,其脾为约,麻子仁丸主之。

麻子仁丸,方:麻子仁二升,芍药半斤,枳实一斤,大黄一斤(去皮),厚朴一尺(去皮),杏仁一升(去皮尖,熬,别作脂)。

上六味,末之,炼蜜和丸梧子大,饮服十丸,日三服,渐加,以知为度。

15. A floating and harsh pulse palpated on the fu yang (tarsus) site is significant because "floating" indicates strong gastric Qi and "harshness" accompanies frequent urination. Interaction between floating and harshness leads to constipation, known as pi yue (spleen constriction). Ma-zi-ren-wan (Apricot Seed and Linum Formula) principally treats the condition.

8 liang peony   16 liang rhubarb

16 liang zhi-shi   1 chi (ca. 30 cm) magnolia bark

2 sheng cannabis seeds   1 sheng apricot seeds

Pulverize the ingredients, knead with honey, and make into pills the size of a sterculia seed. Ten pills are taken with water three times daily. Doses are taken until bowel movement occurs.

第十六节　肾著之病,其人身体重,腰中冷,如坐水中,形如水状,反不渴,小便自利,饮食如故,病属下焦,身劳汗出,衣里冷湿,久久得之,腰以下冷痛,腹重如带五千钱,甘草干姜苓术汤主之。

甘草干姜茯苓白术汤方:甘草、白术各二两,干姜、茯苓各四两。

上四味,以水五升,煮取三升,分温三服,腰中即温。

16. Kidney stagnation manifests generalized heaviness, chills in the lumbus with the feeling as though sitting in water, polyuria (due to moistness), an edematous appearance but no thirst, and a normal appetite. It is a disorder of the lower warmer incurred by lengthy wearing of cold, damp underwear soaked with sweat. The patient experiences chilly pains below the waist and a heavy loin (or abdomen) – he feels as though, he is carrying a load of five thousand taels of coins. Gan-jiang-ling-shu-tang (G. H. A. and Licorice Combination) primarily treats the condition.

4 liang hoelen   2 liang atractylodes
4 liang dried ginger   2 liang licorice

Decoct the four herbs in 5 sheng of water until 3 sheng remains and divide into three portions. One portion is taken three times a day. Warmth will return to the loin.

第十七节　肾死脏,浮之坚,按之乱如转丸,益下入尺中者,死。

17. A genuine renal pulse which is firm on light palpation and resembles a turbulently turning ball on heavy palpation – especially on the chill site – portends death.

第十八节　问曰:三焦竭部,上焦竭善噫,何谓也? 师曰:上焦受中焦气未和,不能消谷,故能噫耳。下焦竭,即遗溺失便,其气不和,不能自禁制,不须治,久则愈。

18. The disciples commented:"Deficiency and exhaustion of the Three Portions of Body Cavity: When the Upper Portion of Body Cavity is deficient and exhausted, the patient will belch frequently. Why is this?"

The master responded:"The Upper Portion is nourished by the Middle Portion. When the Stomach (located in the Middle Portion) Vital Energy is out of harmony, cereal cannot be digested. Indigestion causes the belching. When the Lower Portion is deficient and exhausted, enuresis and fecal incontinence will occur due to a disorder of the Vital Energy, which can no longer control stool and urination. No therapy needs to be adopted. The disorder will subside after a period of time."

第十九节　师曰:热在上焦者,因咳为肺痿;热在中焦者,则为坚;热在下焦者,则尿血,亦令淋秘不通;大肠有寒者,多鹜溏;有热者,便肠垢;小肠有寒者,其人下重便血,有热者必痔。

19. The master said: "Fever lodged in the upper Portion of Body Cavity with prolonged coughing causes pulmonary atrophy; fever in the middle Portion of Body Cavity induces solidification; fever in the lower Portion of Body Cavity results in bloody urine and also in urinary dripping and anuria; chills in the colon cause watery stools; fever in the colon results in the excretion of mucus; chills in the small intestine induce tenesmus and bloody stools; and fever in the small intestine causes hemorrhoids."

第二十节　问曰:病有积,有聚,有鬃气,何谓也?

师曰:积者,脏病也,终不移。聚者腑病也,发作有时,展转痛移,为可治。鬃气者,胁下痛,按之则愈,复发为鬃气。诸积大法,脉来细而附骨者,乃积也。寸口,积在胸中;微出寸口;积在喉中;关上,积在脐旁;上关上,积在心下;微下关,积在少腹;尺中,积在气冲,脉出左,积在左;脉出右;积在右;脉两出,积在中央;各以其部处之。

20. The disciples asked: "Would you explain the diseases known as Ji (accumulation), Ju (conglomeration), and Gu Qi (food Qi)?"

The master said:"Ji (accumulation) is a disease of the Zang organs, or solid viscera. It is immovable throughout. Ju(conglomeration) affects the Fu organs or hollow viscera. It brings on regular seizures of migrating pain and is curable. Gu Qi (food Qi) exhibits hypochondrial aching which disappears on pressure but recurs later. The rule for diagnosing all accumulations is to look for a thin and submerged pulse that is palpable only when the fingers press heavily and touch the radial bone. Such a pulse detected on the cun site locates the accumulation in the chest; a little in front of the cun site locates the accumulation in the throat; on the guan site puts the accumulation in the navel; a little ahead of the guan site locates the accumulation beneath the heart; a little behind the guan site places the accumulation in the lower abdomen; on the chi site, the accumulation lies around Qi chon (region of the urinary bladder); only on the left hand puts the accumulation on the left side of the body and only on the right hand, on the right side of the body; a pulse palpable on both hands locates the accumulation in the central area. Accumulations are treated according to location."

痰饮咳嗽病脉证并治第十二

XII.

On Pulse Syndrome Complex and Treatment of Sputum, Stagnancy, and Cough

第一节　问曰:夫饮有四,何谓也? 师曰:有痰饮,有悬饮,有溢饮,有支饮。

1. The disciples asked: "Are there four types of stagnancy?"

The master said: "Sputum stagnancy, dangling stagnancy, overflowing stagnancy, and branch stagnancy are the four types of stagnancy."

第二节　问曰:四饮何以为异? 师曰:其人素盛今瘦,水走肠间,沥沥有声,谓之痰饮。饮后水流在胁下,咳唾引痛,谓之悬饮。饮水流行,归于四肢,当汗出而不汗出,身体疼重,谓之溢饮。咳逆倚息,短气不得卧,其形如肿,谓之支饮。

2. The disciples asked: "What are the differences between the four types?"

The master said: "A normally stalwart individual who has become thin because of water running in the intestines has sputum stagnancy. If after drinking water flows to the hypochondria causing a cough, expectoration, and dragging pain, it is a dangling stagnancy. If after drinking water flows to the four limbs where it cannot be sweated out causing generalized aching and heaviness, it is an overflowing stagnancy. Branch stagnancy manifests bloating and adverse coughing that so torments that the afflicted must rest by lying against the bed because his gasping makes it impossible for him to lie flat."

第三节　水在心,心下坚筑,短气,恶水不欲饮。

3. When water stagnates in the heart, the patient exhibits hardening beneath the heart, gasping, and a loss of the desire to drink water.

第四节　水在肺,吐涎沫,欲饮水。

4. When water stagnates in the lungs, the patient coughs and expectorates copious sputum and wants to drink water.

第五节　水在脾,少气身重。

5. When water stagnates in the spleen, the patient experiences shallow and short breathing and generalized heaviness.

第六节　水在肝,胁下支满,嚏而痛。

6. When water stagnates in the liver, the patient has distention beneath the hypochondria and painful sneezing.

第七节　水在肾,心下悸。

7. When water stagnates in the kidneys, palpitations occur beneath the heart.

第八节　夫心下有留饮,其人背寒冷如手大。

8. When water stagnates beneath the heart, the patient has chills on his back in an area as large as the palm.

第九节　留饮者,胁下痛引缺盆,咳嗽则转甚。

9. Water stagnation with hypochondrial pain that reaches to and affects the clavicular recess grows more severe on coughing.

第十节　胸中有留饮,其人短气而渴;四肢历节痛,脉沉者,有留饮。

10. Water stagnated in the chest manifests gasping, thirst, and joint pain. The pulse is submerged.

第十一节　膈上病痰,满喘咳吐,发则寒热,背痛腰疼,目泣自出,其人振振身剧,必有伏饮。

11. When a water problem occurs above the diaphragm, the patient exhibits chest distention, asthma, coughing, and expectoration of sputum. If chills and fever, back pain, lower backache, tearing, and trembling of the body accompanies an attack, the condition has become hidden water stagnancy.

第十二节　夫病人饮水多,必暴喘满。凡食少饮多,水停心下,甚者则悸,微者短气。脉双弦者寒也,皆大下后善虚,脉偏弦者,饮也。

12. If the patient drinks too much water, he will definitely develop abrupt asthma and become distended. Generally, a person who eats little food but drinks much water has water stagnation beneath the heart. Cardiac palpitations occur in a severe case or shortness of breath in a mild case. A chordal pulse in both wrists after a strong purgation is evidence of internal weakness (emptiness). A chordal pulse in one wrist only indicates partial (unilateral) stagnation of water.

第十三节　肺饮不弦,但苦喘短气。

13. Pulmonary water stagnation may not exhibit a chordal pulse but will nevertheless trigger asthma and gasping.

第十四节　支饮亦喘而不能卧,加短气,其脉平也。

14. A patient with branch stagnation exhibits only asthma, an inability to lie down, and gasping; the condition is just at a stage where he still has a normal pulse.

第十五节　病痰饮者,当以温药和之。

15. Warm drugs treat water stagnancy diseases.

第十六节　心下有痰饮,胸胁支满,目眩,苓桂术甘汤主之。
苓桂术甘汤方:茯苓四两,桂枝、白术各三两,甘草二两。
上四味,以水六升,煮取三升,分温三服,小便则利。

16. Ling-gui-shu-gan-tang (Atractylodes and Hoelen Combination) relieves water stagnancy beneath the heart which manifests thoracocostal distention and dizziness.

4 liang hoelen　　　　　　　　　　　　3 liang atractylodes
3 liang cinnamon with outer bark removed　　2 liang licorice
Decoct the four herbs in 6 sheng of water until only 3 sheng remains; discard the dregs. The

decoction is taken warmed in three equal doses a day. Urinary flow will then increase.

第十七节 夫短气有微饮,当从小便去之,苓桂术甘汤主之。肾气丸亦主之。

17. Shortness of breath with mild water stagnancy has to be eliminated through urination. It requires Ling-gui-zhu-gan-tang（Atractylodes and Hoelen Combination）or Ba-wei-di-huang-wan（Rehmannia Eight Formula）.

第十八节 病者脉伏,其人欲自利,利反快;虽利,心下续坚满,此为留饮欲去故也,甘遂半夏汤主之。

甘遂半夏汤方:甘遂大者三枚,半夏十二枚(以水一升,煮取半升,去滓),芍药五枚,甘草如指大一枚(炙)。

上四味,以水二升,煮取半升,去滓,以蜜半升,和药汁煎取八合,顿服之。

18. A patient with hidden pulse and a tendency to defecate who feels relieved after defecation but continues to have firm distention beneath the heart has stagnant water that is in the process of leaving. The primary treatment for this condition is Gan-sui-ban-xia-tang（Gan-sui and Pinellia Combination）.

3 pcs. large kansui tubers	5 pieces of peony root
12 pcs. pinellia corms decocted in 1 sheng of water until	1 piece of baked licorice the size of a finger
0.5 sheng remains; discard the dregs	

Place the herbs in 2 sheng of. Water and decoct until sheng remains; discard the dregs. Mix the decoction into 0.5 sheng of honey and boil until 8 ge remains. All the mixture is taken in one draft.

第十九节 脉浮而细滑,伤饮。

19. A floating, thin, and slippery pulse portends injury from water stagnancy.

第二十节 脉弦数,有寒饮,冬夏难治。

20. A chordal and quick pulse indicates chill water stagnancy, a condition difficult to treat.

第二十一节 脉沉而弦者,悬饮内痛。

21. A submerged and chordal pulse evidences dangling stagnancy with internal aching.

第二十二节　病悬饮者,十枣汤主之。

十枣汤方：芫花(熬)、甘遂、大戟各等分。

上三味,捣筛,以水一升五合,先煮肥大枣十枚,取九合,去滓,内药末,强人服一钱匕,羸人服半钱,平旦温服之;不下者,明日更加半钱,得快下后,糜粥自养。

22. A patient with dangling stagnancy should take primarily Shi-zao-tang (Jujube Combination).

$$\left.\begin{array}{l}\text{stewed genkwa}\\\text{kan sui}\\\text{euphorbia}\end{array}\right\}\text{an equal amount of each}\qquad\text{10 big jujubes}$$

Pound the drugs in equal doses into powder. Stew ten large dates in one and a half sheng of water until eight ge remain. Filter the decoction and add one and a half qianbi of the powder for a strong patient and one half qianbi for a weak patient. Serve the lukewarm decoction during the day. If there is no stool, increase dose by one half of a qianbi on the next day. Once a loose stool is observed, serve the patient porridge to complete recovery.

第二十三节　病溢饮者,当发其汗,大青龙汤主之,小青龙汤亦主之。

大青龙汤方：麻黄六两(去节),桂枝二两(去皮),甘草二两(炙),杏仁四十个(去皮尖),生姜三两,大枣十二枚,石膏如鸡子大(碎)。

上七味,以水九升,先煮麻黄,减二升,去上沫,内诸药,煮取三升,去滓,温服一升,取微似汗;汗多者,温粉粉之。

小青龙汤方：麻黄(去节)三两,芍药三两,五味子半升,干姜三两,甘草三两(炙),细辛三两,桂枝三两(去皮),半夏半升(洗)。

上八味,以水一斗,先煮麻黄,减二升,去上沫,内诸药,煮取三升,去滓,温服一升。

23. Da-qing-long-tang (Major Blue Dragon Combination) or Xiao-qing-long-tang (Minor Blue Dragon Combination) treats a patient with overflowing stagnancy by inducing sweating.

Major Blue Dragon Combination

6 liang denoded mahuang	40 pcs. apricot seeds with apex and outer skin removed
2 liang cinnamon with outer bark removed	
2 liang baked licorice	12 pcs. jujube fruits mashed gypsum the volume of an egg
3 liang fresh ginger	

Place the mahuang in 9 sheng of water and decoct until 7 sheng remains. Skim off the supernatent foam. Add the other herbs and boil until 3 sheng remains. Discard the dregs. One sheng warmed induces mild perspiration. If the patient sweats copiously, he should dust his body with wen fen.

Minor Blue Dragon Combination

3 liang denoded mahuang

3 liang peony

3 liang dried ginger

3 liang baked licorice

3 liang asarum

3 liang decorticated cinnamon

0.5 sheng schizandra

0.5 sheng washed pinellia

Put mahuang in 10 sheng of water and decoct until the water has been reduced by 2 sheng; skim off the floating foam, add the other herbs, and decoct again until 3 sheng remains. Discard the dregs. One sheng warmed is taken at a time.

第二十四节　膈间支饮,其人喘满,心下痞坚,面色黧黑,其脉沉紧,得之数十日,医吐下之不愈,木防己汤主之。虚者即愈,实者三日复发,复与不愈者。宜木防己汤去石膏加茯苓芒硝汤主之。

木防己汤方:木防己三两,石膏十二枚鸡子大,桂枝二两,人参四两。

上四味,以水六升,煮取二升,分温再服。

木防己去石膏加茯苓芒硝汤方:木防己,桂枝各二两,人参四两,芒硝三合,茯苓四两。

上五味,以水六升,煮取二升,去滓,内芒硝,再微煎,分温再服,微利则愈。

24. Branch stagnancy located at the diaphragm (with symptoms of panting, distention, hypocardiac obstruction and hardening, a dark facial complexion, and a submerged and tense pulse) in a patient who has been suffering for several weeks and has not been cured by the vomiting or purging methods should be treated primarily with Mu-fang-ji-tang (Stephania and Ginseng Combination). A weak type of the condition may heal, but a firm type may recur three days later. The latter should then be treated with Mu-fang-ji-qu-shi-gao-jia-fu-ling-mang-xiao-tang (Stephania, Hoelen, and Mirabilitum Combination).

Stephania and Ginseng Combination

3 liang stephania

12 pieces gypsum (the size of an egg)

2 liang cinnamon

4 liang ginseng

Place the ingredients in 6 sheng of water and decoct until 2 sheng remains. Divide the decoction into two portions. Each portion is taken warmed.

Stephania, Hoelen, and Mirabilitum Combination

2 liang stephania

2 liang cinnamon

4 liang ginseng

4 liang hoelen

3 ge mirabilitum

Decoct all of the ingredients except mirabilitum with 6 sheng of water until 2 sheng remains. Discard the dregs and add mirabilitum. Decoct slightly again. It is taken in two equal portions. The disease heals when slight diarrhea occurs.

第二十五节　心下有支饮,其人苦冒眩,泽泻汤主之。
泽泻汤方:泽泻五两,白术二两。
上二味,以水二升,煮取一升,分温再服。

25. Branch stagnation causing dizziness requires primarily Ze-xie-tang (Alisma Combination).
5 liang alisma　　　　　　　　　　　2 liang atractylodes
Place the herbs in 2 sheng of water and decoct until 1 sheng remains. It is taken in two equal portions warmed.

第二十六节　支饮胸满者,厚朴大黄汤主之。
厚朴大黄汤方:厚朴一尺,大黄六两,枳实四枚。
上三味,以水五升,煮取二升,分温再服。

26. Branch stagnation with thoracic distention should be treated primarily with Hou-pu-da-huang-tang (Magnolia, Rhubarb, and Chih-shih Combination).
1 chi (ca. 30cm) magnolia bark　　　　4 pcs. zhi-shi fruits
6 liang rhubarb
Place the herbs in 5 sheng of water and decoct until 2 sheng remains. Divide into two equal portions, and take each portion warmed twice a day.

第二十七节　支饮不得息,葶苈大枣泻肺汤主之。方见肺痈中。

27. Branch stagnation with gasping allowing no rest should be treated primarily with Ting-li-da-zao-xie-fei-tang (Lepidium and Jujube Combination).

第二十八节　呕家本渴,渴者为欲解,今反不渴,心下有支饮故也,小半夏汤主之。
《千金》云小半夏加茯苓汤。
小半夏汤方:半夏一升,生姜半斤。
上二味,以水七升,煮取一升半,分温再服。

28. Vomiting normally causes thirst; such thirst signifies that the condition is going to be relieved. If the patient is not thirsty, there is branch stagnation beneath the heart and Xiao-ban-xia-tang (Minor Pinellia Combination) should be prescribed.
1 sheng pinellia　　　　　　　　　8 liang fresh ginger
Place the herbs in 7 sheng of water and decoct until 1.5 sheng remains. The decoction is di-

vided and taken in two equal portions warmed.

第二十九节　腹满,口舌干燥,此肠间有水气,己椒苈黄丸主之。

己椒苈黄丸方: 防己、椒目、葶苈(熬)、大黄各一两。

上四味,末之,蜜丸如梧子大,先食饮服一丸,日三服,稍增,口中有津液。渴者加芒硝半两。

29. The symptoms of abdominal distention and dry mouth and tongue are evidence of water vapor within the intestines for which Ji-jiao-li-huang-wan (Stephania and Lepidium Formula) is indicated.

1 liang stephania   1 liang stewed lepidium

1 liang zanthoxylum seed   1 liang rhubarb

Pulverize the four ingredients, knead with honey, and make into pills as large as a sterculia seed. One pill is taken before each meal. The dosage is increased until salivation occurs. For patients with thirst, add 0.5 liang of mirabilitum.

第三十节　卒呕吐,心下痞,膈间有水,眩悸者,小半夏加茯苓汤主之。

小半夏加茯苓汤方: 半夏一升,生姜半斤,茯苓三两。

上三味,以水七升,煮取一升五合,分温再服。

30. The conformation of sudden vomiting, distention beneath the heart, water at the diaphragm, dizziness, and palpitation should be treated essentially with Xiao-ban-xia-jia-fu-ling-tang (Minor Pinellia and Hoelen Combination).

8 liang fresh ginger   1 sheng pinellia

3 liang hoelen

Place the ingredients in 7 sheng of water and decoct until 1.5 sheng remains. Discard the dregs and divide the decoction into two portions. Each portion is taken warmed.

第三十一节　假令瘦人,脐下有悸,吐涎沫而癫眩,此水也,五苓散主之。

五苓散方: 泽泻一两一分,猪苓三分(去皮),茯苓三分,白术三分,桂枝二分(去皮)。

上五味,为末,白饮服方寸匕,日三服,多饮暖水,汗出愈。

31. A thin individual who has palpitation beneath the navel, slobbering, and dizziness has a water problem and needs Wu-ling-san (Hoelen Five Herb Formula).

1 liang and 1 fen alisma   3 fen atractylodes

3 fen polyporus   2 fen cinnamon with outer bark removed

3 fen hoelen

Pound the ingredients into a powder. One fangcunbi of the powder is taken with boiled water three times daily. It is recommended that extra quantities of warm water be drunk. The disease will leave after sweating occurs.

附方：《外台》茯苓饮,治心胸中有停痰宿水,自吐出水后,心胸间虚,气满,不能食,消痰气,令能食。

茯苓、人参、白术各三两,枳实二两,橘皮二两半,生姜四两。

上六味,水六升,煮取一升八合,分温三服,如人行八九里,进之。

Another formula that treats similar conditions is Fu-ling-yin (Hoelen Combination). It alleviates stagnant or stale water in the chest, a sensation of emptiness and distention from gas in the chest after vomiting, and anorexia. This formula dissipates the vapor of stagnant water and restores appetite.

3 liang hoelen	2 liang zhi-shi
3 liang ginseng	2.5 liang citrus peel
3 liang atractylodes	4 liang fresh ginger

Decoct the ingredients in 6 sheng of water until 1.8 sheng remains, discard the dregs, and divide the decoction into three portions. Each portion is taken warmed periodically. Intervals last as long as it takes to walk 8 or 9 li.

第三十二节　咳家其脉弦,为有水,十枣汤主之。

32. A coughing individual with a chordal pulse due to a water problem requires shi-zao-tang (Jujube Combination).

第三十三节　夫有支饮家,咳烦,胸中痛者,不卒死,至一百日或一岁,宜十枣汤。

33. A patient with branch stagnancy who has a cough, vexation, and intrathoracic aching which has not caused sudden death and who has suffered thus for a hundred days or even a year should preferably take Shi-zao-tang (Jujube Combination).

第三十四节　久咳数岁,其脉弱者,可治;实大数者,死;其脉虚者必苦冒,其人本有支饮在胸中故也。治属饮家。

34. A patient with a weak pulse who has coughed for years is curable, but a patient with a forceful, big, and quick pulse is incurable. In the presence of an empty pulse, the patient will experience giddiness because he has branch stagnancy in the chest. The treatment is the same as for

water stagnancy.

第三十五节　咳逆倚息不得卧,小青龙汤主之。

35. Cough and gasping that prevent one from lying down should be treated with Xiao-qing-long-tang (Minor Blue Dragon Combination).

第三十六节　青龙汤下已,多唾,口燥,寸脉沉,尺脉微,手足厥逆,气从小腹上冲胸咽,手足痹,其面翕热如醉状,因复下流阴股,小便难,时复冒者,与茯苓桂枝五味子甘草汤,治其气冲。

苓桂五味甘草汤方:茯苓四两,桂枝四两(去皮),甘草(炙)三两,五味子半升。

上四味,以水八升,煮取三升,去滓,分温三服。

36. If after purgation with Xiao-qing-long-tang (Minor Blue Dragon Combination) the patient hypersalivates and has a dry mouth, a pulse that is submerged on the cun site and minute on the chi site, cold extremities, Qi flushing upward from the lower abdomen to the chest and throat, paralysis of the extremities, an intensely feverish face like a drunkard's, and dysuria with frequent dizziness (when the Qi retreats to the pudendum and thighs), he must be given Ling-gui-wei-gan-tang (Hoelen, Licorice, and Schizandra Combination) to treat the upflushing Qi.

4 liang hoelen	0.5 sheng schizandra
4 liang decorticated cinnamon	3 liang baked licorice

Decoct the four herbs in 8 sheng of water until only 3 sheng remains; discard the dregs. The decoction is taken warmed in three divided doses a day.

第三十七节　冲气即低,而反更咳、胸满者,用桂苓五味甘草汤去桂,加干姜、细辛,以治其咳满。

苓甘五味姜辛汤方:茯苓四两,甘草、干姜、细辛各三两,五味子半升。

上五味,以水八升,煮取三升去滓,温服半升,日三服。

37. If upflushing Qi has been lowered, yet the patient coughs more severely and has thoracic distention, the condition should be treated essentially with Ling-gan-wu-wei-jiang-xin-tang (Hoelen and Asarum Combination).

4 liang hoelen	3 liang asarum
3 liang licorice	0.5 sheng schizandra
3 liang dried ginger	

Place the ingredients in 8 sheng of water and decoct until 3 sheng remains. Discard the dregs. Three sheng warmed is taken three times a day.

第三十八节　咳满即止,而更复渴,冲气复发者,以细辛、干姜为热药也,服之当逐渴,而渴反止者,为支饮也。支饮者法当冒,冒者必呕,呕者复内半夏以去其水。

桂苓五味甘草去桂加姜辛夏汤方:茯苓四两,甘草、细辛、干姜各二两,五味子、半夏各半升。

上六味以水八升,煮取三升,去滓,温服半升,日三服。

38. If now the cough and distention have ceased, but the patient is very thirsty and the flushing Qi recurs, it is because of the hot herbs Xixin (asarum) and Ganjiang (dried ginger). They cause thirst. If the thirst stops, it is due to the presence of branch stagnancy which as a rule induces dizziness. Vertigo so induced causes vomiting. To treat the vomiting, Banxia (pinellia) incorporated into Ling-gan-wu-wei-jiang-xin-tang (Hoelen and Asarum Combination) will eliminate the stagnant water.

4 liang hoelen	2 liang dried ginger
2 liang licorice	0.5 sheng schizandra
2 liang asarum	0.5 sheng pinellia

Decoct the ingredients in 8 sheng of water until 3 sheng remains. Discard the dregs. One-half sheng warmed is taken three times a day.

第三十九节　水去呕止,其人形肿者,加杏仁主之。其证应内麻黄,以其人遂痹,故不内之;若逆而内之者,必厥。所以然者,以其人血虚,麻黄发其阳故也。

苓甘五味加姜辛半夏杏仁汤方:茯苓四两,甘草三两,五味子半升,干姜三两,细辛三两,半夏半升,杏仁半升(去皮尖)。

上七味,以水一斗,煮取三升,去滓,温服半升,日三服。

39. If by now the water has been eliminated and the vomiting has ceased, but the patient still looks edematous, then add Xingren (apricot seed) to the preceding formula to serve as the primary remedy. As a rule of thumb, Mahuang should be incorporated in a formula to treat an edematous condition; however, if the patient has suffered limb paralysis, that herb is not appropriate. The incorporation of mahuang would definitely result in cold extremities because the person's blood is already depleted, and mahuang further dispels yang, leading to a loss of warm Qi and hence cold limbs. Ling-gan-jiang-wei-xin-xia-ren-tang (Hoelen and Schizandra Combination) is needed instead.

4 liang hoelen	0.5 sheng schizandra
3 liang licorice	0.5 sheng pinellia
3 liang dried ginger	0.5 sheng apricot seed
3 liang asarum	

80

Place the ingredients in 10 sheng of water and decoct until 3 sheng remains. Discard the dregs. One-half sheng warmed is taken three times a day.

第四十节　若面热如醉，此为胃热上冲熏其面，加大黄以利之。

苓甘五味加姜辛半杏大黄汤方：茯苓四两，甘草三两，五味子半升，干姜三两，细辛三两，半夏半升，杏仁半升，大黄三两。

40. A feverish face as though intoxicated results from gastric fever flushing up; rhubarb added to the above formula purges the fever. Ling-gan-jiang-wei-xin-xia-ren-huang-tang (Hoelen, Schizandra, and Rhubarb Combination).

4 liang hoelen　　　　　　　　3 liang rhubarb

3 liang licorice　　　　　　　　0.5 sheng schizandra

3 liang dried ginger　　　　　　0.5 sheng pinellia

3 liang asarum　　　　　　　　0.5 sheng apricot seed

Place the ingredients in 10 sheng of water and decoct until 3 sheng remains. Discard the dregs. Half a sheng warmed is taken three times a day.

第四十一节　先渴后呕，为水停心下，此属饮家，小半夏加茯苓汤主之。

41. A patient who initially manifests thirst followed by vomiting has stagnant water beneath the heart and should be treated primarily with Xiao-ban-xia-jia-fu-ling-tang (Minor Pinellia and Hoelen Combination).

1 sheng pinellia　　　　　　　　3 liang hoelen

8 liang fresh ginger

Place the ingredients in 7 sheng of water and decoct until 1.5 sheng remains. Discard the dregs and divide the decoction into two portions. Each portion is taken warmed.

消渴小便不利淋病脉证并治第十三

XIII.

On Pulse Syndrome Complex and Treatment of Polydipsia, Polyuria, and Urinary Stuttering

第一节　厥阴之为病,消渴,气上冲心,心中疼热,饥而不欲食,食即吐蛔,下之利不止。

1. Absolute yin disease manifests polydipsia, Qi flushing up toward the heart, aching and fever in the heart, hunger but no appetite, vomiting of parasitic worms immediately following eating, and incessant diarrhea after purgation.

第二节　寸口脉浮而迟,浮即为虚,迟即为劳,虚则卫气不足,劳则营气竭。

2. A floating and slow pulse on the cunkou site is significant in that the floating indicates weakness and the slowness, overwork. Weakness leads to deficiency of wei (protective) Qi and overwork leads to exhaustion of ying (vascular) Qi.

第三节　趺阳脉浮而数,浮即为气,数即消谷而大坚,气盛而溲数,溲数即坚,坚数相搏,即为消渴。

3. If the fu yang (tarsal) pulse is floating and quick, floating indicates the state of Qi and quickness the digestion of cereals and constipation. Qi exuberance results in frequent urination which causes, in turn, constipation. The consequent interaction between constipation and frequent urination brings on polydipsia.

第四节　男子消渴,小便反多,以饮一斗,小便一斗,肾气丸主之。

4. Polydipsia and polyuria in a man who excretes an amount of urine equal to the volume of

water drunk should be treated primarily with Ba-wei-di-huang-wan (Rehmannia Eight Formula).

第五节　脉浮,小便不利,微热消渴者,宜利小便,发汗,五苓散主之。

5. Wu-ling-san(Hoelen Five Herb Formula) stimulates urination and perspiration in patients with a floating pulse, oliguria, slight fever, and polydipsia.

第六节　渴欲饮水,水入则吐者,名曰水逆,五苓散主之。

6. Hoelen Five Herb Formula treats thirst in a patient who vomits water immediately after he has drunk it. The condition is called water adversity.

第七节　渴欲饮水不止者,文蛤散主之。
文蛤散方:文蛤五两。
上一味,杵为散,以沸汤五合,和服方寸匕。

7. The patient is thirsty. He drinks great quantities of water but his thirst is still not quenched. Wen-ge-san (Meretrix Formula) treats unquenchable thirst.

5 liang meretrix (clam)

Pound the drug into powder. Place one fangcunbi of powder into five ge of boiling water. Serve the medicine when lukewarm.

第八节　淋之为病,小便如粟状,小腹弦急,痛引脐中。

8. In urinary stuttering the urine drips like grains of millet. Tight cramping of the lower abdomen with pain around the navel also occurs.

第九节　趺阳脉数,胃中有热,即消谷引食,大便必坚,小便即数。

9. A quick pulse on the fu yang site signals a fever in the stomach. The symptoms are constipation, polyuria, and hunger quickly following satiation.

第十节　淋家不可发汗,发汗则必便血。

10. A patient with urinary stuttering should not be sweated because perspiring will induce hematuria.

第十一节　小便不利者,有水气,其人苦渴("苦",一本作"若"),栝蒌瞿麦丸主之。

栝蒌瞿麦丸方：栝蒌根二两,茯苓、薯蓣各三两,附子一枚(炮),瞿麦一两。

右五味,末之,炼蜜丸梧子大,饮服三丸,日三服;不知,增至七八丸,以小便利、腹中温为知。

11. Gua-lou-qu-mai-wan (Trichosanthes and Dianthus Formula) treats agonizing thirst and oliguria due to water retention.

2 liang trichosanthes root	1 liang dianthus
3 liang hoelen	1 pc. baked aconite
3 liang dioscorea	

Pulverize the ingredients, knead with honey, and make into pills the size of a sterculia seed. Three pills along with water are taken three times a day. If no effect is observed, the dosage should be increased to seven or eight pills or until the person urinates and feels warmth in the abdomen.

第十二节　小便不利,蒲灰散主之;滑石白鱼散、茯苓戎盐汤并主之。

蒲灰散方：蒲灰七分,滑石三分。

上二味,杵为散,饮服方寸匕,日三服。

滑石白鱼散方：滑石二分,乱发二分(烧),白鱼二分。

上三味,杵为散,饮服方寸匕("方寸"一本作"半钱"),日三服。

茯苓戎盐汤方：茯苓半斤,白术二两,戎盐弹丸大一枚。

上三味,先将茯苓、白术煎成,入戎盐再煎,分温三服。

12. Simple oliguria (without surface or internal symptoms) should be treated primarily with Pu-hui-san (Typha Ash Formula) as well as Hua-shi-bai-yu-san (Talc and Lepisma Formula) or with Fu-ling-jie-yan-tang (Hoelen and Halite Combination).

Typha Ash Formula

7 fen typha ash	3 fen talc

Pound the ingredients into powder. One fangcunbi of the powder is taken with water three times a day.

Talc and Lepisma Formula

2 fen talc	2 fen lepisma
2 fen scorched human hair	

Pulverize the ingredients. Half a cubic tsun is taken with water three times a day.

Hoelen and Halite Combination

8 liang hoelen	1 pc. salt crystal the size of a bullet
2 liang atractylodes	

Decoct the first two ingredients; then add salt and decoct again. The decoction is divided into three portions and each portion taken warmed.

第十三节　渴欲饮水，口干舌燥者，白虎加人参汤主之。

13. A patient with thirst for water and a dry mouth and lips should drink Bai-hu-jia-ren-sheng-tang (Ginsengand Gypsum Combination).

第十四节　脉浮发热，渴欲饮水，小便不利者，猪苓汤主之。

14. A patient with a floating pulse, fever, thirst for water, and oliguria should be treated essentially with Zhu-ling-tang(Polyporus Combination).

水气病脉证并治第十四

XIV.

On Pulse Syndrome Complex and Treatment of Edema

第一节 师曰:病有风水,有皮水,有正水,有石水,有黄汗。风水,其脉自浮,外证骨节疼痛,恶风;皮水,其脉亦浮,外证胕肿,按之没指,不恶风,其腹如鼓,不渴,当发其汗,正水,其脉沉迟。外证自喘;石水,其脉自沉,外证腹满,不喘;黄汗其脉沉迟,身发热,胸满,四肢头面肿,久不愈,必致痈脓。

1. The master said: "Edema are many: wind, skin, orthodox, stone, and yellow sweat. 'Wind water' causes a floating pulse and the external symptoms of arthralgia and anemophobia. 'Skin water' manifests a floating pulse, edematous swelling which sinks on pressure, no anemophobia, and a normal abdomen without distention or thirst. This disease should be treated by inducing sweating. A submerged and slow pulse and asthma as an external symptom characterize 'orthodox water' and a submerged pulse, abdominal distention, and no asthma, 'stone water' 'Yellow sweat' water disease manifests a submerged and slow pulse, generalized fever, chest distention, and swollen arms, legs, head, and face; if untreated for a prolonged period of time, carbuncular pustulation develops."

第二节 脉浮而洪,浮则为风,洪则为气,风气相搏,风强则为隐疹,身体为痒,痒为泄风,久为痂癞;气强则为水,难以俯仰。风气相击,身体洪肿,汗出乃愈,恶风则虚,此为风水;不恶风者,小便通利,上焦有寒,其口多涎,此为黄汗。

2. A floating and surging pulse is significant. Floating implicates wind and surging, Qi. In an interaction between wind and Qi, if the wind overpowers Qi, tiny papular measles (urticaria) appear on the skin with generalized itching. Ultimately scabbing leprosy (impetigo) forms. If Qi overpowers the wind, a water problem develops that makes the afflicted unable to rest (because of coughing and gasping). If the Qi and wind rival each other, a problem known as feng shui (wind-water disease) with the symptom of severe generalized edema occurs. Feng shui calls for sweating. If anemophobia

occurs after sweating, it is due to surface weakness. If anemophobia does not occur but the patient urinates copiously it indicates chills in the upper warmer. If the patient also drivels copiously, the condition is huang han(yellow sweat)disease.

第三节　寸口脉沉滑者,中有水气,面目肿大有热,名曰风水;视人之目窠上微拥,如蚕新卧起状,其颈脉动,时时咳,按其手足上,陷而不起者,风水。

3. A submerged and slippery pulse on the cun site signifies water in the interior of the body of feng-shui (wind-water disease). Additional symptoms of wind-water disease are facial and ocular swelling – especially of the lower eyelids which come to resemble a silkworm arising from sleep – fever, throbbing of the carotid vessels, frequent coughing, and flesh of the limbs that revives very slowly after being pressed.

第四节　太阳病,脉浮而紧,法当骨节疼痛,反不疼,身体反重而酸,其人不渴,汗出则愈,此为风水。恶寒者,此为极虚,发汗得之。渴而不恶寒者,此为皮水。身肿而冷,状如周痹,胸中窒,不能食,反聚痛,暮躁不得眠,此为黄汗。痛在骨节,咳而喘,不渴者,此为脾胀。其状如肿,发汗则愈。然诸病此者,渴而下利,小便数者,皆不可发汗。

4. A person with a greater yang disease with a floating and tense pulse usually experiences joint pain. If instead his body feels heavy and sore, he has no thirst, and sweating cures him, he has wind-water disease. Chillphobia can occur in the very weakened state following sweating. If the patient is thirsty but without chillphobia, he has skin water disease. Yellow sweat disease evidences generalized edema and chills (just like peripheral paralysis), choking in the chest, loss of appetite, chills accumulating and causing pain above the diaphragm, irritation at dusk resulting in insomnia, and aching of the joints. A cough and asthma, but no thirst, means splenic swelling – pi zhang.

Note: By no means should anyone with any of the above diseases be sweated if he or she exhibits thirst along with diarrhea and polyuria.

第五节　里水者,一身面目黄肿,其脉沉,小便不利,故令病水。假如小便自利,此亡津液,故令渴也,越婢加术汤主之。

5. Interior water – yellow swelling all over the body including the face and eyes, a submerged pulse, and oliguriaprimarily requires Yue-pi-jia-shu-tang (Atractylodes Combination). However polyuria which is causing loss of fluids and hence thirst contraindicates this formula.

6 liang mahuang	2 liang licorice
8 liang gypsum	4 liang atractylodes
3 liang fresh ginger	15 pcs. jujube fruits

Decoct mahuang in 6 sheng of water and skim off the floating foam. Add the other herbs and decoct again until 3 sheng remains. Divide into three portions. Each portion is taken warmed. If the patient has anemophobia, add one baked aconite root.

第六节　趺阳脉当伏,今反紧,本自有寒,疝瘕,腹中痛,医反下之,下之即胸满短气。趺阳脉当伏,今反数,本自有热,消谷,小便数,今反不利,此欲作水。

6. The fu yang (tarsal) pulse normally is hidden. A tense fu yang pulse means the patient has had chills, hernia, tumors, and abdominal pain that have been treated with purgation which has resulted in thoracic distention and labored breathing.

A quick fu yang pulse means an existing fever is causing too rapid digestion of food and frequent urination. If the patient has oliguria, edema will develop.

第七节　寸口脉浮而迟,浮脉则热,迟脉则潜,热潜相搏,名曰沉;趺阳脉浮而数,浮脉即热,数脉即止,热止相搏,名曰伏;沉伏相搏,名曰水;沉则络脉虚,伏则小便难,虚难相搏,水走皮肤,即为水矣。

7. A floating and slow pulse on the cun site portends fever as indicated by the floating and submergence of the primordial Qi as indicated by the slowness. Interaction between fever and submerged Qi leads to sinking of the primordial Qi, a condition called "sedimentation." On the other hand, a floating and quick pulse on the fu yang site signifies fever as indicated by the floating and termination of the wei (protective) Qi as indicated by the quickness. Interaction between fever and the terminated Qi leads to dormancy of the wei Qi, a condition called "dormancy." The presence of both kinds of pulse indicates an interaction between sedimentation and dormancy which results in edema. Moreover, sedimentation also signifies depletion of the meridians and vessels, and dormancy, difficulty in urination. An interaction between meridian depletion and urinary difficulty causes water to move in the skin and hence edema.

第八节　寸口脉弦而紧,弦则卫气不行,即恶寒,水不沾流,走于肠间。

8. A chordal and tense pulse on the cun site signifies that the wei (protective) Qi is motionless as indicated by the "chordal" pulse, and that the patient has chillphobia, as indicated by the tenseness. Consequently, water circulates in the intestines instead of following its normal passage.

第九节　少阴脉紧而沉,紧则为痛,沉则为水,小便即难。脉得诸沉,当责有水,身体肿重,水病脉出者死。

9. A tense and submerged lesser yin pulse signifies pain, as indicated by the tenseness, and water, as indicated by the submergence. The person will have difficulty urinating. Whenever a pulse is submerged, the doctor should suspect the presence of a water disease from which the patient will eventually develop bodily swelling and bloating. A pulse that suddenly becomes floating and bottomless in a person with such a water disease who has been treated with yang ascending drugs portends death.

第十节 夫水病人,目下有卧蚕,面目鲜泽,脉伏,其人消渴,病水腹大,小便不利,其脉沉绝者,有水,可下之。

10. A person who is suffering from edema, whose slightly swollen lower eyelids appear like silkworms lying underneath his eyes, who has a glossy complexion and shiny eyes, a hidden pulse, polydipsia, a big belly due to water disease and oliguria, and a submerged and nearly impalpable pulse needs treatment by purgation for he is suffering from edema.

第十一节 问曰:病下利后,渴饮水,小便不利,腹满因肿者,何也? 答曰:此法当病水,若小便自利及汗出者,自当愈。

11. The disciples asked: "Why does thirst with a desire to drink water, oliguria, and abdominal distention sometimes occur after diarrhea?"

The master said: "Because the patient has water disease. It will cure itself with excessive urination and perspiration."

第十二节 心水者,其身重而少气,不得卧,烦而躁,其人阴肿。

12. A person with cardiac edema exhibits generalized heaviness with labored breathing, an inability to lie down, annoyance and irritation, and hydrocele.

第十三节 肝水者,其腹大不能自转侧,胁下腹痛,时时津液微生,小便续通。

13. A person with hepatic edema has a big belly that hinders body movement, hypochondrial and abdominal aching, and irregular salivation and urination.

第十四节 肺水者,其身肿,小便难,时时鸭溏。

14. A person with pulmonary edema suffers from generalized swelling, diminished urination, and frequent bouts of watery diarrhea.

第十五节　脾水者,其腹大,四肢苦重,津液不生,但苦少气,小便难。

15. A person with splenic edema has a big belly, discomfort from limbic heaviness, a dry mouth, labored breathing, and diminished urination.

第十六节　肾水者,其腹大,脐肿腰痛不得溺,阴下湿,如牛鼻上汗,其脚逆冷,面反瘦。

16. A person with renal edema suffers from abdominal enlargement and umbilical swelling, lumbago with an inability to urinate, moisture beneath the genitals like the sweat on the nose of a cow, cold feet, and a thin face.

第十七节　师曰:诸有水者,腰以上肿,当利小便;腰以下肿;当发汗乃愈。

17. The master said: "Edema occurring below the lumbus should be treated with diuresis, whereas edema above the lumbus requires sweating."

第十八节　师曰:寸口脉沉而迟,沉则为水,迟则为寒,寒水相搏。趺阳脉伏,水谷不化,脾气衰则鹜溏,胃气衰则身肿。少阳脉卑,少阴脉细,男子则小便不利,女子则经水不通,经为血,血不利则为水,名曰血分。

问曰:病有血分水分,何也?

师曰:经水前断,后病水,名曰血分,此病难治;先病水,后经水断,名曰水分,此病易治。何以故? 去水,其经自下。

18. The master said: "A submerged and slow pulse on the cun site is evidence of water, as indicated by the submergence, and chills, as indicated by the slowness. Here water and chills are in interaction. A hidden pulse on the fu yang (tarsal) site should alert the doctor to indigestion reflecting splenic deterioration that leads to diarrhea and eventually gastric deterioration. Generalized edema soon follows. Consequently, the patient develops a submerged and weakened lesser yang pulse or a thin lesser yin pulse. Oliguria occurs in the male and amenorrhea in the female. Amenorrhea also results in edema of xue fen, a blood disease."

The disciples asked: "Edema may be caused by a blood disorder or by pathogenetic Water. How can they be differentiated?"

The master replied: "In female patients, if amenia appears before edema, it is a case of edema caused by blood disorder and quite difficult to treat. If edema appears before amenia, case is one of edema caused by water-evil and thus is easily treated. Why then? First disperse the stagnant Water;

then menstruation will resume."

第十九节　问曰：病者苦水，面目身体四肢皆肿，小便不利，脉之，不言水，反言胸中痛，气上冲咽，状如炙肉，当微咳喘，审如师言，其脉何类？

师曰：寸口脉沉而紧，沉为水，紧为寒，沉紧相搏，结在关元，始时尚微；年盛不觉，阳衰之后，营卫相干，阳损阴盛，结寒微动，肾气上冲，喉咽塞噎，胁下急痛。医以为留饮而大下之，气击不去，其病不除；后重吐之，胃家虚烦，咽燥欲饮水，小便不利，水谷不化，面目手足浮肿；又与葶苈丸下水，当时如小差，食饮过度，肿复如前，胸胁苦痛，像若奔豚，其水扬溢，则浮咳喘逆。当先攻击冲气，令止，乃治咳，咳止，其喘自差。先治新病，病当在后。

19. The disciples asked: "What type of pulse would a person have who suffers from oliguria and edema in the face, eyes, limbs, and body and who complains of chest pain and flushing of Qi to the throat as if a piece of barbecued meat were stuck there? Also when, on taking the pulse, you do not diagnose a water problem, but instead confront a mild cough and asthma?"

The master replied: "If the pulse on the cun site is sub-merged and tense, the submergence signifies water and the tenseness, chills. Initially, interaction between water and chills results in accumulation of the two at the guan yuan (lower abdomen) area three inches below the navel; usually the condition is mild and undetectable by the person himself because of his youthfulness. However, as yang degenerates, the intravascular and extra-vascular systems begin to interfere with each other. Yang becomes subjugated and yin becomes exuberant. The chills begin to agitate slightly causing renal Qi to flush and choke the throat and acute pain to arise under the ribs. The doctor may mistake the condition for water stagnancy and prescribe a strong purgative.

"It will not help but in fact will cause the Qi to remain in place. The doctor may then ignorantly treat this condition with a strong emetic which will cause gastric weakness and annoyance, a dry throat with a desire to drink water, oliguria, indigestion, and edema of the face, arms, and legs. For this, the doctor may administer Ting-Li-wan (Lepidium Formula) to induce diuresis. This will relieve the symptoms somewhat but if the person later eats excessively, his abdomen will again swell as before, his chest and ribs will ache so severely that he will act like a fleeing hog, and the water will well up and overflow causing coughing and adverse asthma. Treatment is to attack the flushing of Qi first and to treat the cough only after the Qi has stopped flushing. When the coughing stops, the asthma will ameliorate spontaneously. The rule of treatment to follow is: Treat the new disease first, then the old one."

第二十节　风水，脉浮，身重，汗出恶风者，防己黄芪汤主之，腹痛者加芍药。

20. A person with wind-water disease exhibiting a floating pulse, generalized heaviness, perspiring, and anemophobia should take primarily Fang-ji-huang-qi-tang (Stephania and Astragalus

Combination). If the patient also has abdominal aching, add shaoyao (peony) to the formula.

第二十一节　风水恶风，一身悉肿，脉浮不渴，续自汗出，无大热，越婢汤主之。

越婢汤方：麻黄六两，石膏半斤，生姜三两，甘草二两，大枣十五枚。

上五味，以水六升，先煮麻黄，去上沫，内诸药，煮取三升，分温三服，恶风者加附子一枚炮；风水加术四两。

21. A person with wind-water disease exhibiting anemophobia, generalized edema, a floating pulse, lack of thirst, continuous spontaneous perspiring, and an absence of high fever needs primarily Yue-pi-tang (Mahuang and Gypsum Combination).

6 liang mahuang	2 liang licorice
8 liang gypsum	15 pcs. jujube fruits
3 liang fresh ginger	

Decoct mahuang in 6 sheng of water. Skim off the supernatent foam, then add the other ingredients and decoct until 3 sheng remains. Divide the decoction into three portions. Each portion is taken warmed. If the patient also has anemophobia, add one baked aconite root. If he has wind-water disease, add 4 liang of atractylodes.

第二十二节　皮水为病，四肢肿，水气在皮肤中，四肢聂聂动者，防己茯苓汤主之。

防己茯苓汤方：防己三两，黄芪三两，桂枝三两，茯苓六两，甘草二两。

上五味，以水六升，煮取二升，分温三服。

22. A skin water disease exhibiting swelling of the extremities, water in the skin, and trembling limbs should be treated primarily with Fang-ji-fu-ling-tang (Stephania and Hoelen Combination).

3 liang stephania	6 liang hoelen
3 liang astragalus	2 liang licorice
3 liang cinnamon	

Place the ingredients in 6 sheng of water and decoct until 2 sheng remains. The decoction is divided into three portions. Each portion is taken warmed.

第二十三节　里水，越婢加术汤主之，甘草麻黄汤亦主之。

越婢加术汤方：方见上。于内加白术四两。

甘草麻黄汤方。甘草二两，麻黄四两。

上二味，以水五升，先煮麻黄，去上沫，内甘草，煮取三升，温服一升，重复汗出，不汗，再服，慎风寒。

23. A skin water disease can be treated primarily with Yue-pi-jia-shu-tang (Atractylodes Combination) as well as Gan-cao-ma-huang-tang (Licorice and Mahuang Combination).

2 liang licorice   4 liang mahuang

Decoct mahuang in 5 sheng of water, skim off the foam, then add licorice and decoct again until one sheng remains. Cover the patient with a heavy quilt to promote sweating. If sweating does not occur, give one more dose. Care should be taken to prevent contraction of chills from a draft or the cold.

第二十四节　水之为病,其脉沉小,属少阴;浮者为风,无水虚胀者,为气。水,发其汗即已,脉沉者宜麻黄附子汤,浮者宜杏子汤。

麻黄附子汤方:麻黄三两,甘草二两,附子一枚(炮)。

上三味,以水七升,先煮麻黄,去上沫,内诸药,煮取二升半,温服八分,日三服。

杏子汤方:方未见。

24. Edema that evidences a submerged and thin pulse is of the lesser yin type, but a floating pulse signifies a wind disease. When there is no water but just empty distention, the patient has a Qi disease. Sweating cures a water disease; Ma-huang-fu-zi-tang (Mahuang and Aconite Combination) is for persons with a sumberged pulse and Xing-zi-tang (Apricot Seed Combination) for those with a floating pulse.

Mahuang and Aconite Combination

3 liang mahuang   1 pc. baked aconite root

2 liang licorice

Decoct mahuang in 7 sheng of water. After removing the foam, add the other ingredients and decoct until 2.5 sheng remains. Divide the decoction into three portions. Each is taken warmed three times a day.

Apricot Seed Combination

4 liang mahuang   50 pcs. apricot seeds

2 liang baked licorice

Decoct mahuang in 7 sheng of water until the decoction has reduced by 2 sheng, then skim off the floating foam and add the other ingredients. Decoct again until 3 sheng remains and remove the dregs. One sheng warmed is taken. When perspiration occurs, the subsequent doses are suspended.

第二十五节　厥而皮水者,蒲灰散主之。

25. Pu-hui-san (Typha Ash Formula) treats primarily a skin-water disease with chills.

第二十六节　问曰:黄汗之为病,身体肿,发热汗出而渴,状如风水,汗沾衣,色正黄如柏汁,脉自沉,何从得之?

师曰:以汗出入水中浴,水从汗孔入得之,宜芪芍桂酒汤主之。

黄芪芍药桂枝苦酒汤方:黄芪五两,芍药三两,桂枝三两。

上三味,以苦酒一升,水七升,相和,煮取三升,温服一升,当心烦,服至六七日乃解,若心烦不止者,以苦酒阻故也。

26. The disciples asked: "Yellow sweat disease brings on generalized swelling (or heaviness), fever, perspiring with thirst, an appearance resembling wind-water disease, sweat resembling phellodendron juice that stains the clothes with a yellow color, and a submerged pulse. How does one get this disease?"

The master said: "If a person bathes while perspiring, water invades the pores and causes yellow sweat." The disease should be treated primarily with Huang-qi-shao-yao-gui-zhi-ku-jiu-tang (Astragalus, Peony, and Cinnamon Combination).

5 liang astragalus   3 liang cinnamon

3 liang peony

Place the herbs in a mixture of one sheng of vinegar and 7 sheng of water and decoct until 3 sheng remains. One sheng is taken warmed. Discomfort in the heart can be relieved by taking the decoction for six to seven days. If the annoyance has not been relieved by then, the vinegar is obstructing the treatment.

第二十七节　黄汗之病,两胫自冷;假令发热,此属历节;食已汗出,又身常暮卧盗汗出者,此劳气也;若汗出已反发热者,久久其身必甲错,发热不止者,必生恶疮;若身重,汗出已辄轻者,久久必身瞤,瞤即胸中痛,又从腰以上必汗出,下无汗,腰髋弛痛,如有物在皮中状,剧者不能食,身疼重,烦躁,小便不利,此为黄汗,桂枝加黄芪汤主之。

桂枝加黄芪汤方:桂枝、芍药各三两,甘草二两,生姜三两,大枣十二枚,黄芪二两。

上六味,以水八升;煮取三升,温服二升,须臾饮热稀粥一升余,以助药力,温服以微汗;若不汗,更服。

27. Yellow sweat disease often causes chilling of the tibia. Tibial fever, on the other hand, is an arthritic condition. If a patient perspires after eating, sleeps at dusk, and has night sweats, he is suffering from fatigue and Qi exhaustion. If he perspires but still has a fever, he will eventually develop horny and coarse skin. If the fever persists, noxious sores arise.

A person with generalized heaviness who feels relieved after sweating will eventually experience trembling, an aching chest on trembling, perspiration above the waist only, laxness with an aching of the waist and hips, and a sensation as though something were under his skin. Severe episodes will render the patient unable to eat and cause a heavy feeling, vexation and irritation, and oliguria. This type of yellow sweat disease requires treatment primarily with Gui-zhi-jia-huang-qi-tang (Cinnamon and Astragalus Combination).

3 liang cinnamon	3 liang fresh ginger
3 liang peony	2 liang astragalus
2 liang licorice	12 pcs. jujubes

Place the herbs in 8 sheng of water and decoct until 3 sheng remains. One sheng is taken warmed, followed a short while later by a little more than one sheng of hot, thin rice congee to promote the drug's effect. Cover the patient in warm clothes or a quilt to induce mild sweating. If the patient does not perspire, more of the decoction should be taken.

第二十八节　师曰:寸口脉迟而涩,迟则为寒,涩为血不足;趺阳脉微而迟,微则为气,迟则为寒。寒气不足,则手足逆冷,手足逆冷,则营卫不利,营卫不利,则腹满肠鸣相逐;气转膀胱,营卫俱劳;阳气不通即身冷,阴气不通即骨疼;阳前通则恶寒,阴前通则痹不仁;阴阳相得,其气乃行,大气一转,其气乃散,实则失气,虚则遗尿,名曰气分。

28. The master said: "In a slow and harsh pulse on the cun site, the slowness indicates chills and the harshness, blood insufficiency. Likewise, a minute and slow pulse on the fu yang (tarsal) site indicates Qi insufficiency and chills respectively. Chills and Qi insufficiency lead to adverse chilling of the arms and legs which in turn hinders the functioning of the intravascular and extra vascular systems resulting in alternating abdominal distention and borborygmus, interference in the functioning of the urniary bladder, and ultimately, exhuastion of both the intravascular and extravascular systems. Obstructed yang Qi produces generalized chilling while obstructed yin Qi produces aching bones. If yang moves alone, chills occur; if yin moves alone, abdominal distention and paralysis arise. Only when yang and yin go together will the Qi move normally. Once the grand(universal) Qi turns, the chills will disperse through the passage of gas in a firm conformation and enuresis in a weak conformation. Since the condition involves Qi, it is named Qi fen."

第二十九节　气分,心下坚大如盘,边如旋杯,水饮所作,桂枝去芍药加麻辛附子汤主之。

桂枝去芍药加麻黄细辛附子汤方:桂枝三两,生姜三两,甘草二两,大枣十二枚,麻黄、细辛各二两,附子一枚(炮)。

上七味,以水七升,煮麻黄,去上沫,内诸药,煮取二升,分温三服,当汗出,如虫行皮中,即愈。

29. Qi fen manifests as subcardiac hardening as large as a dish, the rim of which feels like a turning cup. Stagnant water(converted from the chilled Qi) is the cause and Gui-zhi-qu-shao-yao-jia-ma-huang-xi-xin-fu-zi-tang (Cinnamon, Mahuang, Asarum, and Aconite Combination) is the primary treatment.

3 liang cinnamon	2 liang licorice
3 liang fresh ginger	12 pcs. jujubes
2 liang mahuang	1 pc. baked aconite
2 liang asarum	

Place mahuang in 7 sheng of water and decoct. Skim off the supernatent foam. Add the other herbs and decoct again until 2 sheng remains. Divide the decoction into three portions. It is taken warmed. The patient will perspire and feel as though insects are crawling within his skin. This sensation portends recovery.

第三十节　心下坚大如盘，边如旋盘，水饮所作，枳术汤主之。

枳术汤方：枳实七枚，白术二两。

上二味，以水五升，煮取三升，分温三服，腹中软，即当散也。

30. Subcardiac hardening as large as a dish, the rim of which feels like a turning dish indicates stagnant water. Zhi-shu-tang(Zhi-shi and Atractylodes Combination) is the primary treatment.

7 pcs. zhi-shi fruits	2 liang atractylodes

Place the ingredients in 5 sheng of water and decoct until 3 sheng remains. Divide the decoction into three portions. One portion warmed is taken at a time. Softening of the abdomen reflects dispersion of the stagnant water and of the subcardiac hardening, too.

附方：

《外台》防己黄芪汤：治风水脉浮，为在表，其人或头汗出，表无他病，病者但下重，从腰以上为和，腰以下当肿及阴，难以屈伸。方见风湿中。

Fang-ji-huang-qi-tang (Stephania and Astragalus Combination) also treats wind-water disease with a floating pulse signifying a surface condition. The patient may perspire on his head only and have no other surface symptoms. There is heaviness below the waist but all is normal above the waist. The swelling from the waist down to the pudendum causes difficulty in flexing and extending.

黄疸病脉证并治第十五

XV.

On Pulse Syndrome Complex and Treatment of Jaundice

第一节　寸口脉浮而缓,浮则为风,缓则为痹,痹非中风,四肢苦烦,脾色必黄,瘀热以行。

1. A floating and moderate pulse on the cun site signifies evil wind, as indicated by the floating, and paralysis, as indicated by the moderateness. However, paralysis is not due to wind stroke alone, but rather to evil wind and moisture converting into fever. The arms and legs feel distressed and vexed and the skin turns yellowish when a moist fever that was formerly stagnated in the spleen circulates throughout the body.

第二节　趺阳脉紧而数,数则为热,热则消谷;紧则为寒,食即为满。尺脉浮为伤肾;趺阳脉紧为伤脾。风寒相搏,食谷即眩,谷气不消,胃中苦浊,浊气下流,小便不通,阴被其寒,热流膀胱,身体尽黄,名曰谷疸。

额上黑,微汗出,手足中热,薄暮即发,膀胱急,小便自利,名曰女劳疸,腹如水状不治。心中懊侬而热,不能食,时欲吐,名曰酒疸。

2. A tense and quick pulse on the fu yang (tarsal) site signifies fever and quick digestion of food, as indicated by the quickness, and chills, hence gastric distention after eating, as indicated by the tenseness. A floating pulse on the chi site denotes injury to the kidneys, and a tense pulse on the fu yang site, injury to the spleen. Interaction between evil wind and chills hinders clear Qi from ascending and as a consequence promotes dizziness after eating, indigestion, stressful disturbance in the stomach, descending of turbid Qi, blocked urine flow, chills in the spleen, fever flowing into the urinary bladder, and a generalized yellowing. This is called gu dan (cereal jaundice). On the other hand, darkening along the temples, slight perspiration, feverish hands and feet at dusk, cystic cramps, and frequent urination characterize a condition known as nü lao dan (jaundice due to sexual overindulgence and fatigue). The presence of a swollen abdomen as in edema denotes an incurable

condition. If the patient feels discomfort, stress, and heat in his heart and has a loss of appetite along with nausea, he is suffering from jiu dan (wine jaundice).

第三节　阳明病,脉迟者,食难用饱,炮则发烦,头眩,小便必难,此欲作谷疸。虽下之,腹满如故,所以然者,脉迟故也。

3. A person with a slow pulse who is suffering from sunlight yang disease will find it hard to eat his fill, feel vexation and giddiness after eating, and urinate with difficulty. These symptoms indicate oncoming gu dan (cereal jaundice). Even if a purgative is taken, the abdomen remains swollen because of the slow pulse.

第四节　夫病酒黄疸,必小便不利,其候心中热,足下热,是其证也。

4. Patients with jiu dan disease (wine jaundice) have decreased urine secretion and fever in the heart and in the soles of their feet.

第五节　酒黄疸者,或无热,靖言了了,腹满欲吐,鼻燥。其脉浮者;先吐之,沉弦者先下之。

5. A patient with wine jaundice may not have a fever and may be perfectly calm with lucid speech but at the same time have abdominal distention, nausea, and sometimes a dry nose. In this situation, induce vomiting if the pulse is floating or purgation if the pulse is submerged and chordal.

第六节　酒疸,心中热,欲吐者,吐之愈。

6. A patient with wine jaundice who experiences fever in his heart and feels nauseated may be cured by vomiting.

第七节　酒疸下之,久久为黑疸,目青面黑,心中如啖蒜齑状,大便正黑,皮肤、爪之不仁,其脉浮弱,虽黑微黄,故知之。

7. Wine jaundice mistreated by purgation eventually becomes dark jaundice. Dark circles under the eyes, a dark complexion, a sensation in the heart like that that occurs after eating garlic, black stools, skin numbness to scratching, a floating and weak pulse, and slightly yellowish skin with a dark background, all these symptoms appear.

第八节　师曰:病黄疸,发热,烦喘、胸满、口燥者,以病发时,火劫其汗,两热所得,然黄家所得,从湿得之,一身尽发热而黄,肚热,热在里,当下之。

8. The master said: "The reason why jaundice exhibits fever, annoyance and stridor, chest distention, and dry mouth is that at the onset of the disease fire evil acting together with the fever is expelling sweat. As a rule, fire evil and fever disperse each other, but jaundice occurs here because moisture combines with the fever. If the patient has an internal abdominal fever, he should be purged."

第九节 脉沉,渴欲饮水,小便不利者,皆发黄。

9. In the presence of a submerged pulse, thirst with a desire to drink water, and oliguria, there will be jaundice.

第十节 腹满,舌痿黄,躁不得睡,属黄家。

10. Abdominal distention, withering and yellowing of the body, and irritability causing insomnia characteristically accompany jaundice.

第十一节 黄疸之病,当以十八日为期,治之十日以上瘥,反剧者为难治。

11. Jaundice runs a course of eighteen days. Generally, it disappears after ten days of treatment; after that if aggravated it will prove difficult to cure.

第十二节 疸而渴者,其疸难治;疸而不渴者,其疸可治;发于阴部,其人必呕;阳部,其人振寒而发热也。

12. Jaundice accompanied by thirst does not respond to treatment while jaundice without thirst does. If the disease derives from the yin (interior), the patient will definitely vomit; if from the yang (surface), he will shiver with fever.

第十三节 谷疸之为病,寒热不食,食即头眩,心胸不安,久久发黄,为谷疸,茵陈蒿汤主之。
茵陈蒿汤方:茵陈蒿六两,栀子十四枚,大黄二两。
上三味,以水一斗,先煮茵陈,减六升,内二味,煮取三升,去滓,分温三服。小便当利,尿如皂角汁状,色正赤。一宿腹减,黄从小便去也。

13. Chills and fever which cause anorexia, dizziness after eating, and discomfort in the heart

and chest portend gu dan(cereal jaundice). The afflicted primarily needs Yin-chen-hao-tang (Capillaris Combination).

6 liang capillaris   14 pcs. gardenia fruits

2 liang rhubarb

Place the capillaris in 10 sheng of water and decoct until 6 sheng remains; add the other two herbs and decoct the mixture again until 3 sheng remains; discard the dregs. Divide the decoction into three portions. One portion warmed is taken each time. Urinary volume will definitely increase after taking the decoction, and the urine will have a red tint like gleditschia juice. The abdomen will reduce overnight because the jaundice toxin is discharging through the urine.

第十四节　黄家,日晡所发热,而反恶寒,此为女劳得之;膀胱急,少腹满,身尽黄,额上黑,足下热,因作黑疸;其腹胀如水状,大便必黑,时溏,此女劳之病,非水也。腹满者难治,硝石矾石散主之。

硝石矾石散方:硝石、矾石(烧)等分。

上二味,为散,以大麦粥汁和服方寸匕,日三服。病随大小便去,小便正黄,大便正黑,是候也。

14. If a person with jaundice develops a fever with chillphobia at dusk, he has nü lao (sexual exhaustion), characterized further by an urgency to urinate, abdominal distention, and yellow skin. These symptoms together with a darkening around the temples and fever in the soles of the feet signify dark jaundice. Edema-like abdominal distention, black stools, and frequent diarrhea indicate nü lao rather than edema. A patient with nü lao accompanied by abdominal distention is difficult to cure. He requires Xiao-shi-fan-shi-san (Niter and Alum Formula).

niter   burnt alum

equal amounts of each

Pulverize the ingredients and mix one fangcunbi of the powder in a congee prepared from barley. The congee is eaten three times daily. The disease toxins will be discharged in the form of yellow urine and black feces.

第十五节　酒黄疸,心中懊侬或热痛,栀子大黄汤主之。

栀子大黄汤方:栀子十四枚,大黄一两,枳实五枚,豉一升。

上四味,以水六升,煮取二升,分温三服。

15. A patient suffering from wine jaundice with annoyance and heart stress, or fever and aching, primarily requires Zhi-zi-da-huang-tang (Gardenia and Rhubarb Combination).

14 pcs. gardenia fruits   1 liang rhubarb

5 pcs. zhi-shi fruits   1 sheng soya bean relish

Place the ingredients in 6 sheng of water and decoct until 2 sheng remains. Divide the decoction into three portions. Each portion is taken warmed.

第十六节　诸病黄家,但利其小便;假令脉浮,当以汗解之,宜桂枝加黄芪汤主之。

16. Diuresis relieves various kinds of jaundice. If the patient exhibits a floating pulse, the condition should be treated by inducing sweating. Therefore, it is appropriate to treat primarily with Gui-zhi-jia-huang-qi-tang (Cinnamon and Astragalus Combination).

第十七节　诸黄,猪膏发煎主之。
猪膏发煎方:猪膏半斤,乱发如鸡子大三枚。
上二味,和膏中煎之,发消药成,分再服。病从小便出。

17. Zhu-gao-fa-jian-fang (Lard and Human Hair Combination) also treats various kinds of jaundice.

8 liang lard　　　　　　　　　　3 balls human hair, each ball the size of an egg

Decoct both ingredients until the hair dissolves completely. Divide the decoction into two portions. One portion is taken twice a day. The disease will discharge through the urine.

第十八节　黄疸病,茵陈五苓散主之。
茵陈五苓散方:茵陈蒿末十分,五苓散五分。方见痰饮中。
上二物和,先食饮方寸匕,日三服。

18. Yin-chen-wu-ling-san (Capillaris and Hoelen Formula) is also a primary treatment for jaundice.

10 fen capillaris powder　　　　　　　5 fen Wu-ling-san

Mix together the two ingredients. One fangcunbi of the mixture is taken before meals three times daily.

第十九节　黄疸腹满,小便不利而赤,自汗出,此为表和里实,当下之,宜大黄硝石汤。
大黄硝石汤方:大黄、黄柏、硝石各四两,栀子十五枚。
上四味,以水六升,煮取二升,去滓内硝,更煮取一升,顿服。

19. Jaundice with abdominal distention, scanty red urine, and spontaneous perspiring characterizes a harmonized surface and firm interior. Purgation with Da-huang-xiao-shi-tang (Rhubarb and Niter Combination) should be instituted.

4 liang rhubarb　　　　　　　　　　4 liang niter

4 liang phellodendron   15 pcs. gardenia fruits

Put all ingredients except niter in 6 sheng of water and decoct until 2 sheng remains. Discard the dregs, add niter, and decoct again until one sheng remains. The decoction is taken in one draft.

第二十节   黄疸病,小便色不变,欲自利,腹满而喘,不可除热,除热必哕,哕者,小半夏汤主之。

20. Fever-purging formulas given to patients with jaundice who have normal colored urine, a tendency to urinate frequently, and abdominal distention with asthma will cause retching. Xiao-Ban-xia-tang (Minor Pinellia Combination) treats retching.

第二十一节   诸黄,腹痛而呕者,宜小柴胡汤。

21. Xiao-chai-hu-tang(Minor Bupluerum Combination) treats various jaundice conditions with vomiting and abdominal aching.

柴胡半斤,黄芩三两,人参三两,甘草三两,半夏半斤,生姜三两,大枣十二枚。
上七味,以水一斗二升,煮取六升,去滓,再煎取三升,温服一升,日三服。

8 liang bupleurum   0.5 sheng pinellia

3 liang scute   3 liang fresh ginger

3 liang ginseng   12 pcs. jujube fruits

3 liang licorice

Decoct the ingredients with 12 sheng of water until 6 sheng remains. Discard the dregs and decoct again until 3 sheng remains. One sheng warmed is taken three times daily.

第二十二节   男子黄,小便自利,当与虚劳小建中汤。

22. The tonic Xiao-jian-zhong-tang (Minor Cinnamon and Peony Combination) treats jaundice in a man who urinates frequently.

Two other formulas that treat jaundice are given below.

《千金》麻黄醇酒汤:治黄疸。
麻黄三两。
上一味,以美清酒五升,煮取二升半,顿服尽。冬月用酒、春月用水煮之。

Mahuang-chun-jiu-tang（Mahuang and Wine Combination）treats jaundice.

3 liang mahuang

Place the single herb in 5 sheng of fine clear wine and decoct until 2.5 sheng remains. All the formula is taken in one draft. In winter, decoct with wine; in spring, decoct with water.

瓜蒂散，治诸黄。

Gua-di-san（Melon Pedicel Combination）treats various kinds of jaundice.

20 pcs. melon pedicels

Shred and decoct the pedicels in one sheng of water until 0.5 sheng remains; discard the dregs and take the decoction in one draft.

惊悸吐衄下血胸满瘀血病脉证并治第十六

XVI.

On Pulse Syndrome Complex and Treatment of Convulsions and Palpitation, Hematemesis, Nosebleeds, Hematochezia, Chest Fullness and Blood Stasis

第一节　寸口脉动而弱,动即为惊,弱则为悸。

1. Pulse on the cunkou site is fluttering and weak. Fluttering pulse indicates convulsions. Weak pulse indicates palpitations.

第二节　师曰:尺脉浮,目睛晕黄,衄未止,晕黄去,目睛慧了,知衄今止。

2. The master said: "A floating pulse on the chi site and yellowish eyes accompany a nosebleed. The ocular yellowing will fade and the eyes clear when the bleeding ceases."

第三节　又曰:从春至夏衄者太阳,从秋至冬衄者阳明。

3. The master further said: "Nosebleeds that occur during spring and summer are of the greater yang whereas those that occur in autumn and winter are of the sunlight yang."

第四节　衄家不可汗,汗出必额上陷,脉紧急,直视不能眴,不得眠。

4. A patient with a nosebleed should not be sweated because his temples will sink and he will develop a tense and quick pulse, a fixed stare, and insomnia.

第五节　病人面无色,无寒热。脉沉弦者,衄;浮弱,手按之绝者,下血;烦咳者,必吐血。

5. A pallid complexion, absence of chills and fever, and a submerged and chordal pulse accompany a nosebleed. If the pulse feels floating and weak, dying out upon heavy palpation, it is a sign of hemorrhage. If the patient exhibits vexation and coughing besides, he will soon vomit blood.

第六节　夫吐血,咳逆上气,其脉数而有热,不得卧者,死。

6. A patient who vomits blood and has an adverse cough, flushing up of qi, a quick pulse, and fever and thus an inability to lie down will die.

第七节　夫酒客咳者,必致吐血,此因极饮过度所致也。

7. An alcoholic with a cough will definitely soon begin to vomit blood as a consequence of the overdrinking of alcohol.

第八节　寸口脉弦而大,弦则为减,大则为芤,减则为寒,芤则为虚,寒虚相搏,此名曰革,妇人则半产漏下,男子则亡血。

8. The pulse is tight and huge on the cunkou. When pressed deeply, it is not as strong as a true tight pulse. Though huge, it is void within. Such pulse is called "leathery" (void-tight). Tight pulse of reduced strenght indicates prevalence of pathogenetic Cold. Void pulse reflects Interior Deficiency. When void-tight pulse occurs in female patients, this indicates premature delivery or mild, chronic bloody vaginal discharge. In male patients, it indicates loss of blood and sperm.

第九节　亡血不可发其表,汗出即寒栗而振。

9. A patient who has lost blood should not be treated with sudorifics because after perspiring he will experience chills and trembling.

第十节　病人胸满,唇痿,舌青,口燥,但欲漱水,不欲咽,无寒热,脉微大来迟,腹不满,其人言我满,为有瘀血。

10. Evidences of stagnant blood are chest fullness; thin lips; a bluish tongue; dry mouth with a desire to rinse with, but not swallow, water; absence of chills and fever; a minute, big, and slow pulse; and no abdominal distention though the patient feels bloated.

第十一节　病者如热状,烦满,口干燥而渴,其脉反无热,此为阴伏,是瘀血也,当下之。

11. When a patient feels feverish and has annoyance and distention with a dry mouth and a sensation of thirst but a pulse that indicates the absence of fever, he has hidden yin and stagnant blood; he should be treated by purgation.

第十二节　火邪者,桂枝去芍药加蜀漆牡蛎龙骨救逆汤主之。

桂枝救逆汤方：桂枝三两(去皮),甘草二两(炙),生姜三两,牡蛎五两(熬),龙骨四两,大枣十二枚,蜀漆三两(洗去腥)。

上为末,以水一斗二升,先煮蜀漆,减二升,内诸药,煮取三升,去滓,温服一升。

12. Gui-zhi-qu-shao-yao-jia-shu-qi-mu-li-long-gu-jiu-ni-tang (Cinnamon, Dichroa Sprout, Dragon Bone, and Oyster Shell Combination) treats those suffering from evil fire.

3 liang cinnamon	4 liang dragon bone
2 liang licorice	12 pcs. jujube fruits
3 liang fresh ginger	3 liang dichroa sprouts washed until free from
5 liang stewed oyster shell	fish odor

Pulverize the first six ingredients, decoct dichroa sprouts in 12 sheng of water until 10 sheng remains, add the other ingredients, and decoct again until 3 sheng remains. Discard the dregs. One sheng warmed is taken each time.

第十三节　心下悸者,半夏麻黄丸主之。

半夏麻黄丸方：半夏、麻黄等分。

右二味,末之,炼蜜和丸小豆大,饮服三丸,日三服。

13. A patient with palpitation beneath the heart primarily needs Ban-xia-ma-huang-wan (Pinellia and Mahuang Formula).

pinellia	mahuang
equal amounts of each	

Pulverize the ingredients, knead with honey, and make into pills, each the size of a small bean. Three pills are taken with water three times daily.

第十四节　吐血不止者,柏叶汤主之。

柏叶汤方：柏叶、干姜各三两,艾三把。

右三味,以水五升,取马通汁一升,合煮取一升,分温再服。

14. A person who incessantly vomits blood should immediately take Bo-ye-tang (Biota Leaves Combination).

3 liang biota leaves   3 handfuls moxa

3 liang dried ginger

Decoct the three ingredients in 5 sheng of water and 1 sheng of horse urine until 1 sheng remains. Divide into two portions. Each portion is taken warmed twice a day.

第十五节　下血,先便后血,此远血也,黄土汤主之。

黄土汤方：甘草、干地黄、白术、附子(炮)、阿胶、黄芩各三两,灶中黄土半斤。

上七味,以水八升,煮取三升,分温二服。

15. Huang-tu-tang（Fuolung-kan Combination）treats "distal blood," bleeding in which first stool, then blood is evacuated. Chi-xiao-dou-dang-gui-san（Phaseolus and Dang-gui Formula）treats "proximal blood," bleeding in which first blood, then stool is evacuated.

Huang-tu-tang

3 liang licorice   3 liang gelatin

3 liang dried rehmannia   3 liang scute

3 liang atractylodes   8 liang yellow earth from the kitchen stove

3 liang baked aconite

Decoct the ingredients in 8 sheng of water until 3 sheng remains. Divide the decoction into two portions. Each portion is taken warmed twice a day.

第十六节　心气不足,吐血衄血,泻心汤主之。

泻心汤方：亦治霍乱。大黄二两,黄连、黄芩各一两。

上三味,以水三升,煮取一升,顿服之。

16. Xie-xin-tang（Coptis and Rhubarb Combination）treats a patient with deficiency of heart qi, hematemesis, and nosebleeds.

2 liang rhubarb   1 liang scute

1 liang coptis

Decoct the ingredients in 3 sheng of water until one sheng remains. It is taken in one draft.

呕吐哕下利病脉证治第十七

XVII.

On Pulse Syndrome Complex and Treatment of Nausea and Vomiting, Retching and Diarrhea

第一节　夫呕家,有痈脓,不可治呕,脓尽自愈。

1. A person who vomits out carbuncular pus should not undergo treatment with the antiemesis method since the condition will heal spontaneously as the pus depletes.

第二节　先呕却渴者,此为欲解;先渴却呕者,为水停心下,此属饮家;呕家本渴,今反不渴者,以心下有支饮故也,此属支饮。

2. Vomiting followed by thirst signals recovery. Thirst followed by vomiting means stagnant water under the heart. A patient who vomits is usually thirsty. The absence of thirst means there is branch stagnation beneath the heart.

第三节　问曰:病人脉数,数为热,当消谷引食,而反吐者,何也? 师曰:以发其汗,令阳微,膈气虚,脉乃数,数为客热,不能消谷,胃中虚冷故也。脉弦者虚也,胃气无余,朝食暮吐,变为胃反,寒在于上,医反下之,令(今)脉反弦。故名曰虚。

3. The disciples asked: "A patient with a quick indicative of fever ought to be able to digest food quickly. What does it mean if he regurgitates food?"

The master said: "Regurgitation occurs as a consequence of being treated by the sweating method which has diminished yang and weakened diaphragm Qi. The quick characteristic of the pulse, denotes affliction by a 'guest' fever. The inability to digest food occurs because the stomach has been weakened and chilled. A chordal pulse indicates depletion of gastric Qi. Consequently food eaten in the morning will be vomited undigested in the evening. It occurs when a doctor purges a chill downward that was formerly lodged in the upper warmer. The condition is due to, and known as, weakness."

第四节　寸口脉微而数,微则无气,无气则营虚,营虚则血不足,血不足则胸中冷。

4. A minute and quick pulse on the cun site signifies a lack of Qi and hence blood weakness. Blood weakness leads to blood deficiency which in turn causes chills in the chest.

第五节　趺阳脉浮而涩,浮则为虚,涩则伤脾,脾伤则不磨,朝食暮吐,暮食朝吐,宿谷不化,名曰胃反,脉紧而涩,其病难治。

5. A floating and harsh pulse on the fu yang site is significant in that the floating denotes weakness, and the harshness, splenic injury. An injured spleen does not digest food. Consequently, morning food is vomited in the evening, and evening food the next morning – a condition known as "gastric adversity" (regurgitation). If the condition exhibits a tense and harsh pulse, it is difficult to cure.

第六节　病人欲吐者,不可下之。

6. A patient with nausea should not be purged.

第七节　哕而腹满,视其前后,知何部不利,利之即愈。

7. Depending on whether there is a problem with urination or defecation, diuresis or catharsis can heal retching and abdominal distention.

第八节　呕而胸满者,茱萸汤主之。
茱萸汤方:吴茱萸一升,人参三两,生姜六两,大枣十二枚。
上四味,以水五升,煮取三升,温服七合,日三服。

8. Wu-zhu-yu-tang (Evodia Combination) treats vomiting with chest distention.

| 1 sheng evodia | 3 liang ginseng |
| 12 pcs. jujube fruits | 6 liang fresh ginger |

Decoct the ingredients in 5 sheng of water until 3 sheng remains. 0.7 sheng warmed is taken three times daily.

第九节　干呕,吐涎沫,头痛者,茱萸汤主之。

9. Evodia Combination also treats dry heaves, frothy salivation, and headache.

第十节 呕而肠鸣,心下痞者,半夏泻心汤主之。

半夏泻心汤方:半夏半升(洗),黄芩三两,干姜三两,人参三两,黄连一两,大枣十二枚,甘草(炙)二两。

上七味,以水一斗,煮取六升,去滓,再煮取三升,温服一升,日三服。

10. Ban-xia-xie-xin-tang (Pinellia Combination) treats vomiting accompanied by borborygmus and obstruction beneath the heart.

0.5 sheng washed pinellia	1 liang coptis
2 liang scute	2 liang baked licorice
3 liang dried ginger	12 pcs. jujube fruits
3 liang ginseng	

Place the ingredients in 10 sheng of water and decoct until 6 sheng remains. Discard the dregs and decoct the contents again until 3 sheng remains. One sheng warmed is taken three times daily.

第十一节 干呕而利者,黄芩加半夏生姜汤主之。

黄芩加半夏生姜汤方:黄芩三两,甘草二两(炙),芍药二两,半夏半升,生姜三两,大枣十二枚。

上六味,以水一斗,煮取三升,去滓,温服一升,日再,夜一服。

11. Huang-qin-jia-ban-xia-sheng-jiang-tang (Scute, Pinellia, and Ginger Combination) treats dry heaves with diarrhea.

3 liang scute	0.5 sheng pinellia
2 liang baked licorice	3 liang fresh ginger
1 liang peony	12 pcs. jujube fruits

Place all ingredients in 10 sheng of water and decoct until 3 sheng remains. Discard the dregs. One sheng warmed is taken twice in the daytime and once at night.

第十二节 诸呕吐,谷不得下者,小半夏汤主之。

12. Xiao-ban-xia-tang (Minor Pinellia Combination) alleviates various conditions of vomiting in which ingested food can not enter the stomach.

第十三节 呕吐而病在隔上,后思水者,解,急与之,思水者,猪苓散主之。

猪苓散方:猪苓、茯苓、白术各等分。

上三味,杵为散,饮服方寸匕,日三服。

13. When the cause of the disease is located above the diaphragm and vomiting followed by a desire to drink water occurs, it means that the patient is going to recover. A little water should be given immediately. Zhu-ling-san (Polyporus Formula) slakes excessive thirst.

polyporus   atractylodes

hoelen

equal amounts of each

Pulverize the ingredients. One fangcunbi of the powder is taken mixed in boiled water three times daily.

第十四节　呕而脉弱,小便复利,身有微热,见厥者,难治,四逆汤主之。

四逆汤方:附子(生用)一枚,干姜一两半,甘草二两(炙)。

上三味,以水三升,煮取一升二合,去滓,分温再服。强人可大附子一枚,干姜三两。

14. Si-ni-tang (Aconite, Ginger, and Licorice Combination) relieves vomiting, a weak pulse, frequent urination, and slight generalized fever in a person with chills. The condition is difficult to cure.

1 raw aconite root   1.5 liang dried ginger

2 liang baked licorice

Decoct the ingredients in 3 sheng of water until 1.2 sheng remains, discard the dregs, and divide into two portions. Each portion is taken warmed. For strong patients, use a large aconite root and 3 liang of dried ginger.

第十五节　呕而发热者,小柴胡汤主之。

小柴胡汤方:柴胡半斤,黄芩三两,人参三两,甘草三两,半夏半斤,生姜三两,大枣十二枚。

上七味,以水一斗二升,煮取六升,去滓,再煎取三升,温服一升,日三服。

15. A patient with vomiting and fever should be treated primarily with Xiao-chai-hu-tang (Minor Bupleurum Combination).

8 liang bupleurum   0.5 sheng pinellia

3 liang scute   3 liang fresh ginger

3 liang ginseng   12 pcs. jujube fruits

3 liang licorice

Decoct the ingredients with 12 sheng of water until 6 sheng remains. Discard the dregs and decoct again until 3 sheng remains. One sheng warmed is taken three times daily.

第十六节　胃反呕吐者,大半夏汤主之。《千金》云:"治胃反不受,食入即吐。"《外台》云:"治呕食,心下痞鞕者。"

大半夏汤方:半夏二升(洗完用),人参三两,白蜜一升。

上三味,以水一斗二升,和蜜扬之二百四十遍,煮药,取二升半,温服一升余分再服。

16. Da-ban-xia-tang(Pinellia, Ginseng, and Mel Combination) relieves regurgitation of undigested food.

2 sheng washed pinellia　　　　　　　3 liang ginseng

1 sheng white honey

Blend the herbs into a mixture of the honey and 12 sheng of water 240 times, using a special motion in which the material is scooped up and allowed to drop through the air, then decoct until 2.5 sheng remains. One sheng warmed is taken for the first dose. The remaining part is divided into two portions and each portion taken individually.

第十七节　食已即吐者,大黄甘草汤主之。

大黄甘草汤方:大黄四两,甘草一两。

上二味,以水三升,煮取一升,分温再服。

17. A patient who vomits immediately after eating a meal should take primarily Da-huang-gan-cao-tang (Rhubarb and Licorice Combination).

4 liang rhubarb　　　　　　　　　　1 liang licorice

Place the herbs in 3 sheng of water and decoct until one sheng remains. Divide the decoction into two portions. Each portion is taken warmed.

第十八节　胃反吐而渴,欲饮水者,茯苓泽泻汤主之。

茯苓泽泻汤方:茯苓半斤,泽泻四两,甘草二两,桂枝二两,白术三两,生姜四两。

上六味,以水一斗,煮取三升,内泽泻,再煮取二升半,温服八合,日三服。

18. A patient with regurgitation and thirst and a desire to drink water should take Fu-ling-ze-xie-tang (Hoelen, Alisma, and Ginger Combination).

8 liang hoelen　　　　　　　　　　　2 liang cinnamon

4 liang alisma　　　　　　　　　　　3 liang atractylodes

2 liang licorice　　　　　　　　　　　4 liang fresh ginger

Decoct the herbs except alisma in 10 sheng of water until 3 sheng remains; add alisma and decoct again until 2.5 sheng remains. 8 ge warmed is taken three times daily.

第十九节　吐后,渴欲得水而贪饮者,文蛤汤主之。兼主微风、脉紧、头痛。

文蛤汤方：文蛤五两，麻黄、甘草、生姜各三两，石膏五两，杏仁五十枚，大枣十二枚。

上七味，以水六升，煮取二升，温服一升，汗出即愈。

19. A patient who craves water and drinks gluttonously due to thirst after vomiting should take Wen-ge-tang (Meretrix Combination). The formula also treats wind illnesses with a tense pulse and headache.

5 liang meretrix (clams)	5 liang gypsum
3 liang mahuang	50 pcs. apricot seeds
3 liang licorice	12 pcs. jujube fruits
3 liang fresh ginger	

Place all the ingredients in 6 sheng of water and decoct until 2 sheng remains. One sheng warmed is taken. Perspiring heals the condition.

第二十节　干呕吐逆，吐涎沫，半夏干姜散主之。

半夏干姜散方：半夏、干姜各等分。

上二味，杵为散，取方寸匕，浆水一升半，煮取七合，顿服之。

20. Ban-xia-gan-jiang-san (Pinellia and Ginger Formula) relieves dry heaves, regurgitation, and frothy salivation.

pinellia	dried ginger

equal amounts of each

Pound the ingredients into powder; decoct one fangcunbi of the powder in 1.5 sheng of soil water until 0.7 sheng remains. It is taken all at one draft.

第二十一节　病人胸中似喘不喘，似呕不呕，似哕不哕，彻心中愦愦然无奈者，生姜半夏汤主之。

生姜半夏汤方：半夏半升，生姜汁一升。

上二味，以水三升，煮半夏，取二升，内生姜汁，煮取一升半，小冷，分四服，日三夜一服；止，停后服。

21. Sheng-jiang-ban-xia-tang (Fresh Ginger and Pinellia Combination) helps a patient who experiences an indescribable nauseous feeling and discomfort in the heart, sensations in his chest similar to asthma, vomiting, or retching, but has none of these ailments.

0.5 sheng pinellia	1 sheng fresh ginger juice

Decoct pinellia in 3 sheng of water until 2 sheng remains; add fresh ginger juice and decoct again until 1.5 sheng remains. After slight cooling, divide into four portions. It is taken three times during the day and once at night. When the symptoms disappear, treatment can be suspended.

第二十二节　干呕哕,若手足厥者,橘皮汤主之。

橘皮汤方:橘皮四两,生姜半斤。

上二味,以水七升,煮取三升,温服一升,下咽即愈。

22. Ju-pi-tang (Aurantium Combination) relieves dry heaves and retching along with cold extremities.

4 liang citrus peel　　　　　　　　　　8 liang fresh ginger

Decoct the ingredients in 7 sheng of water until 3 sheng remains. One sheng at a time is taken warmed. Upon swallowing the formula, the disease should leave.

第二十三节　哕逆者,橘皮竹茹汤主之。

橘皮竹茹汤方:橘皮二升,竹茹二升,人参一两,甘草五两,生姜半斤,大枣三十枚。

上六味,以水一斗,煮取三升,温服一升,日三服。

23. A patient with adverse retching should take Ju-pi-zhu-ru-tang (Aurantium and Bamboo Combination).

2 sheng citrus, peel　　　　　　　　　5 liang licorice

2 sheng bamboo taenia　　　　　　　　8 liang fresh ginger

1 liang ginseng　　　　　　　　　　　30 pcs. jujube fruits

Decoct the ingredients in 10 sheng of water until 3 sheng remains. One sheng warmed is taken three times daily.

第二十四节　夫六腑气绝于外者,手足寒,上气脚缩;五脏气绝于内者,利不禁;下甚者,手足不仁。

24. When the vitality of the six hollow viscera is exhausted on the surface of the body, the extremities become cold, Qi flushes, and the feet cramp. When the vitality of the five solid viscera is exhausted in the interior of the body, incessant diarrhea occurs. If severe, the diarrhea causes the limbs to become numb.

第二十五节　下利,脉沉弦者下重,脉大者为未止,脉微弱数者为欲自止,虽发热不死。

25. In the presence of diarrhea, a submerged and chordal pulse indicates a grave condition; a big pulse, a condition that yet has no sign of cessation; and a minute, weak, and quick pulse, one wherein the diarrhea is going to cease and the patient will live in spite of a fever.

第二十六节　下利,手足厥冷,无脉者,炙之不温;若脉不还,反微喘者,死;少阴负趺阳者,为顺也。

26．A patient with diarrhea, cold arms and legs, and a hidden pulse will die if his body does not warm, his pulse does not revive, and he nevertheless has asthma after treatment with moxibustion. A hidden lesser yin pulse with a palpable fu yang(tarsal) pulse means the patient is recovering.

第二十七节　下利有微热而渴,脉弱者,今自愈。

27．A patient with diarrhea, mild fever, thirst, and a weak pulse is recovering spontaneously.

第二十八节　下利,脉数,有微热汗出,今自愈;设脉紧,为未解。

28．A patient who is perspiring and has diarrhea, a mild fever, and a quick pulse is recovering spontaneously; but if the pulse is tense, he is not recovering yet.

第二十九节　下利,脉数而渴者,今自愈;设不差,必清(圊)脓血,以有热故也。

29．A patient with diarrhea, a quick pulse, and thirst is recovering spontaneously; if not, a fever will cause the discharge of purulent and bloody stool.

第三十节　下利,脉反弦,发热身汗者,自愈。

30．A patient who is suffering from diarrhea and yet exhibits a chordal pulse, fever, and generalized sweating is recovering spontaneously.

第三十一节　下利气者,当利其小便。

31．The rendering of diuresis treats a patient with diarrhea and discharge of gas.

第三十二节　下利,寸脉反浮数,尺中自涩者,必清(圊)脓血。

32．A patient with diarrhea and a floating and quick pulse on the cun site and a harsh one on the chi site will discharge purulent and bloody stools.

第三十三节　下利清谷,不可攻其表,汗出必胀满。

33. Diarrhea containing undigested food should not be treated by the surface attack method because it will bring forth abdominal distention after perspiration.

第三十四节　下利脉沉而迟,其人面少赤,身有微热,下利清谷者,必郁冒,汗出而解,病人必微热。所以然者,其面戴阳,下虚故也。

34. A patient suffering from lientery with a submerged and slow pulse, a slightly ruddy complexion, and mild generalized fever will feel giddy. Sweating relieves the condition. However, before sweating the patient will experience mild chills and facial hyperemia due to weakness of the lower warmer.

第三十五节　下利后脉绝,手足厥冷,晬时脉还,手足温者生,脉不还者死。

35. A patient with cold limbs and interruption of pulse after diarrhea will not die, if the pulse revives after a period of time equivalent to one cycle of circulation and if his limbs become warm, but he will die if the pulse does not revive.

第三十六节　下利腹胀满,身体疼痛者,先温其里,乃攻其表,温里宜四逆汤,攻表宜桂枝汤。

36. A patient with diarrhea, distention of the abdomen, and generalized aching should be treated by first warming the interior before attacking the surface symptoms. Si-ni-tang(Aconite, Ginger, and Licorice Combination) warms the interior while Gui-zhi-tang (Cinnamon Combination) attacks surface symptoms.

第三十七节　下利,三部脉皆平,按之心下坚者,急下之,宜大承气汤。

37. A patient with diarrhea, normal pulses on the three sites cun, guan, and chi, and hardening beneath the heart as detected by palpation should be purged immediately with Da-cheng-qi-tang (Major Rhubarb Combination) as the preferred formula.

第三十八节　下利,脉迟而滑者,实也。利未欲止,急下之,宜大承气汤。

38. Diarrhea with a slow and slippery pulse signifies a firm condition of the stomach. If the diarrhea shows no sign of ceasing, the person should be purged immediately with Da-cheng-qi-tang

（Major Rhubarb Combination）as the preferred formula.

第三十九节　下利，脉反滑者，当有所去，下乃愈，宜大承气汤。

39. In diarrhea a slippery pulse signifies that purging will cure the patient. The remedy called for is Da-cheng-qi-tang(Major Rhubarb Combination）as the preferred formula.

第四十节　下利已差，至其年月日时复发者，以病不尽故也，当下之，宜大承气汤。

40. A patient who suffers from a recurrence of diarrhea one year later on the same hour, same day, and same month needs to be purged with Major Rhubarb Combination（see above）as the preferred formula because his disease has not been eradicated yet.

第四十一节　下利谵语者，有燥屎也，小承气汤主之。小承气汤方：大黄四两　厚朴三两（炙），枳实大者三枚（炙）。
上三味，以水四升，煮取一升二合，去滓，分温二服，得利则止。

41. Xiao-cheng-qi-tang（Minor Rhubarb Combination）treats a patient with delirium following diarrhea. This signifies the presence of dry stool.

4 liang rhubarb   3 pcs. large baked zhi shi fruits

3 liang seared magnolia bark

Decoct the ingredients with 4 sheng of water until 1.2 sheng remains. Discard the dregs and divide the decoction into two portions. A portion is taken until a bowel movement occurs.

第四十二节　下利，便脓血者，桃花汤主之。
桃花汤方：赤石脂一斤（一半剉，一半筛末），干姜一两，粳米一升。
上三味，以水七升，煮米令熟，去滓，温七合，内赤石脂末方寸匕，日三服。若一服愈，余勿服。

42. Tao-hua-tang（Kaolin and Oryza Combination）treats a patient with diarrhea of purulent, bloody stools.

8 liang red bole, one-half shredded, the other half pulverized and sieved

1 liang dried ginger

1 sheng non-sticky rice

Place the three ingredients, not including the powdered half of red bole, in 7 sheng of water and decoct until the rice is well cooked. Discard the dregs. Seven-tenths sheng warmed, together with one fangcunbi of the powdered red bole, are taken three times daily. If the disease disappears after one treatment, the remaining doses need not be taken.

第四十三节　热利下重者,白头翁汤主之。

白头翁汤方:白头翁二两,黄连、黄柏、秦皮各三两。

上四味,以水七升,煮取二升,去滓,温服一升;不愈更服。

43. A patient with feverish and severe diarrhea should take Bai-tou-weng-tang (Anemone Combination).

3 liang anemone	3 liang phellodendron
3 liang coptis	3 liang fraxinus

Decoct the ingredients in 7 sheng of water until 2 sheng remains. After discarding the dregs one sheng is taken warmed; if no effect is observed, the dose should be repeated.

第四十四节　下利后更烦,按之心下濡者,为虚烦也,栀子豉汤主之。

栀子豉汤方:栀子十四枚,香豉四合(绵裹)。

上二味,以水四升,先煮栀子,得二升半,内豉,煮取一升半,去滓,分二服,温进一服,得吐则止。

44. If after a bout of diarrhea the patient feels more vexed and has softness beneath the heart when palpated, it means weakness vexation which should be treated primarily with Zhi-zi-chǐ-tang (Gardenia and Soya Combination).

14 pcs. gardenia fruits wrapped in linen　　　4 ge soya bean relish

Decoct the gardenia in 4 sheng of water until 2.5 sheng remains. Add the relish and decoct again until 1.5 sheng remains. Discard the dregs. The decoction is divided into two portions and one portion warmed is taken at a time until vomiting occurs.

第四十五节　下利清谷,里寒外热,汗出而厥者,通脉四逆汤主之。

通脉四逆汤方:附子大者一枚(生用),干姜三两(强人可四两),甘草二两(炙)。

右三味,以水三升,煮取一升二合,去滓,分温再服。

45. A patient with lientery, internal chills and external fever, and perspiration and chilling needs Tong-mai-si-ni-tang (Aconite, Ginger, and Licorice Combination Fortified).

1 large raw aconite　　　3 liang dried ginger (4 liang for stronger patients)

2 liang baked licorice

Decoct the ingredients in 3 sheng of water until 1.2 sheng remains. Discard the dregs. The decoction is divided into two portions and each portion taken warmed.

第四十六节　下利,肺痛,紫参汤主之。
紫参汤方:紫参半斤,甘草三两。
上二味,以水五升,先煮紫参,取二升,内甘草,煮取一升半,分温三服。

46. Zi-sheng-tang (Zi sheng Combination) primarily treats diarrhea accompanied with "lung ache".

8 liang zi-sheng 　　　　　　　　　　　3 liang licorice

Decoct Zi sheng first in 5 sheng of water until 2 sheng remains. Add the licorice and decoct again until 1.5 sheng remains. Divide into three portions. Each portion is taken warmed.

第四十七节　气利,诃梨勒散主之。
诃梨勒散方:诃梨勒十枚(煨)。
上一味,为散,粥饮和,顿服。

47. Ke-li-le-san (Terminalia Formula) treats Qi diarrhea.

10 pcs. toasted terminalia fruits

The fruit is toasted and pulverized and taken together with rice congee in one draft.

Two other formulas treat similar conditions.

《外台》黄芩汤:治干呕下利。
黄芩、人参、干姜各二两,桂枝一两,大枣十二枚,半夏半斤。
上六味,以水七升,煮取三升,温分三服。

Huang-qin-tang (Scute Combination) treats retching and diarrhea.

2 liang scute 　　　　　　　　　　　1 liang cinnamon

2 liang ginseng 　　　　　　　　　　12 pcs. jujubes

2 liang dried ginger 　　　　　　　　0.5 sheng pincllia

Decoct the ingredients in 7 sheng of water until 3 sheng remains. Divide the decoction into three portions. Each portion is taken warmed.

《千金翼》小承气汤:治大便不通,哕,数谵语。

Xiao-cheng-qi-tang (Minor Rhubarb Combination) treats constipation, retching, and frequent delirium.

疮痈肠痈浸淫病脉证并治第十八

XVIII.
On Pulse Syndrome Complex and
Treatment of Sores, Carbuncles,
Intestinal Carbuncles and Spreading Effusive Sores

第一节 诸浮数脉,应当发热,而反洒淅恶寒,若有痛处,当发其痈。师曰:诸痈肿,欲知有脓无脓,以手掩肿上,热者为有脓,不热者为无脓。

1. A person with a floating and quick pulse usually has a fever. However, if instead he has chillphobia and a feeling of aching, he is developing carbunculosis.

The master said: "To tell whether pus has formed or not in the carbuncle swellings, cover the swelling with your hand. If the area feels hot, there is pus; if not, there is no pus."

第二节 肠痈之为病,其身甲错,腹皮急,按之濡如肿状,腹无积聚,身无热,脉数,此为肠内有痈脓,薏苡附子败酱散主之。

薏苡附子败酱散方:薏苡仁十分 附子二分 败酱五分。

上三味,杵为末,取方寸匕,以水二升,煎减半,顿服,小便当下。

2. Generalized scaly skin, tense abdominal skin with a tumid softness when pressed, the absence of abdominal tumors and generalized fever, and a quick pulse portend intestinal carbuncular pustulation. Treatment primarily calls for Yi-yi-fu-zi-bai-jiang-san (Coix, Aconite, and Thlaspi Formula).

10 fen coix   5 fen thlaspi

2 fen aconite

Pound the ingredients into powder and decoct one fangcunbi of the powder with 2 sheng of water until the volume reduces by half. The decoction is taken in one draft.

第三节 肠痈者,小腹肿痞,按之即痛,如淋,小便自调,时时发热,自汗出,复恶寒;其脉迟紧者,脓未成,可下之,当有血;脉洪数者,脓已成。不可下也,大黄牡丹汤主之。

大黄牡丹汤方:大黄四两,牡丹一两,桃仁五十个,瓜子半斤,芒硝三合。

上五味,以水六升,煮取一升,去滓,内芒硝,再煎沸,顿服之,有脓当下;如无脓,当下血。

3. Lower abdominal swelling and hardening with aching upon pressure like that of urinary stuttering, normal urination, frequent fever, spontaneous sweating, and chillphobia characterize intestinal carbuncles. A slow and tense pulse indicates that pus has not yet developed. The condition may be treated by purgation which will cause bleeding. If the patient's pulse is surging and quick, pus has developed and the condition should not be treated by purgation but with Da-huang-mu-dan-tang (Rhubarb and Moutan Combination).

4 liang rhubarb
0.5 sheng benincasa seeds
1 liang moutan
3 ge mirabilitum
50 pcs. persica seeds

Decoct all ingredients except the mirabilitum in 6 sheng of water until one sheng remains. Discard the dregs, add the mirabilitum, and bring to a boil. The decoction is taken warmed in one draft. If pus is present in the body, it will be discharged; if there is none, blood will be discharged.

第四节 问曰:寸口脉浮微而涩,然当亡血,若汗出,设不汗者云何? 答曰:若身有疮,被刀斧所伤,亡血故也。

4. The disciples asked: "A floating, minute, and harsh pulse on the cun site accompanies a loss of blood or profuse sweating. However, if the patient is not perspiring what is his condition?"

The master answered: "The patient might have a knife wound that has caused a loss of blood."

第五节 病金疮,王不留行散主之。

王不留行散方:王不留行十分(八月八日采),蒴藋细叶十分(七月七日采),桑东南根白皮十分(三月三日采),甘草十八分,川椒三分(除目及闭口,去汗),黄芩二分,干姜二分,厚朴二分,芍药二分。

上九味,桑根皮以上三味烧灰存性,勿令灰过,各别杵筛,合治之为散,服方寸匕,小疮即粉之,大疮但服之,产后亦可服。如风寒,桑东根勿取之。前三物皆阴干百日。

5. Wang-bu-liu-xing-san (Vaccaria Formula) treats knife wounds.

10 fen saponaria harvested on the eighth day of the eighth month according to the lunar calendar

10 fen tiny leaves of sambucus harvested on the seventh day of the seventh month according to

the lunar calendar

10 fen white bark of roots of mulberry growing easterly or southerly, harvested on the third day of the third month according to the lunar calendar

3 fen baked zanthoxylum, exclude the black seeds and closed carpels, then bake to expel the oil

18 fen licorice	2 fen magnolia bark
2 fen scute	2 fen peony
2 fen dried ginger	

Char the first three ingredients in a way that preserves their original nature, do not burn. Pound them and the remaining herbs into powder and pass the powder through a fine sieve. One fangcunbi is taken each time. For small wounds, apply the powder directly on the site. For large wounds, the powder is taken orally. The formula also aids puerperal women. Easterly growing mulberry roots should not be harvested on windy and chilly days. The first three herbs should be dried in the shade for one hundred days.

Two other formulas expel pus and resolve toxicity and carbuncles.

排脓散方：枳实十六枚,芍药六分,桔梗二分。
上三味,杵为散,取鸡子黄一枚,以药散与鸡黄相等,揉和令相得,饮和服之,日一服。

Pai-nong-san (Platycodon and Zhi-shi Formula)

16 pcs. zhi-shi fruits	6 fen peony
2 fen platycodon	

Pound the ingredients into powder. Mix one egg yolk with an equal amount of the powder. Blend the mixture till homogeneous and take it with boiled water three times a day.

排脓汤方：甘草二两,桔梗三两,生姜一两,大枣十枚。
上四味,以水三升,煮取一升,温服五合,日再服。

Pai-nong-tang (Platycodon and Jujube Combination)

2 liang licorice	1 liang fresh ginger
3 liang platycodon	10 pcs. jujube fruits

Decoct the ingredients in 3 sheng of water until one sheng remains. Half a sheng warmed is taken twice daily.

第六节　浸淫疮,从口流向四肢者可治;从四肢流来入口者不可治。

6. Chronic spreading, effusive sores that start in the mouth and spread towards the arms and

legs are curable whereas sores that begin on the extremities and spread to the mouth are incurable.

第七节 浸淫疮，黄连粉主之。

7. Huang-lian-fen (Coptis Powder) treats chronic, spreading effusive sores.

跌蹶手指臂肿转筋阴狐疝蚘虫病脉证第十九

XIX.

On Pulse Syndrome Complex and Treatment of Tarsal Collapse; Swelling and Spasms of the Fingers, Hands, and Arms; Hernias; and Infestations with Worms

第一节　师曰:病跌蹶,其人但能前,不能却,刺腨入二寸,此太阳经伤也。

1. The master said: "A person with tarsal collapse can only move forward and not backward; he should be treated by inserting (acupuncture) needles into the calf at a depth of two cun (inches) because that is the path of the greater yang meridian."

第二节　病人,常以手指臂肿动,此人身体瞤瞤者,藜芦甘草汤主之。藜芦甘草汤方: 方未见。

2. Li-lu-gan-cao-tang (Veratrum and Licorice Combination) soothes a patient with trembling swollen fingers and arms and general trembling. (The contents of this formula do not appear in the original text)

第三节　转筋之为病,其人臂脚直,脉上下行,微弦,转筋入腹者,鸡屎白散主之。
鸡屎白散方: 鸡屎白。
上一味,为散,取方寸匕,以水六合,和,温服。

3. Spasms cause the back and feet to become rigidly straight and the pulse to become long, minute, and chordal. If the spasms advance to the abdomen, the patient needs Ji-shi-bai-san (Chicken Feces Powder).

a sufficient amount of white matter of chicken feces

Pulverize the feces and mix one fangcunbi of the powder with 6 he of water. The solution is taken warmed.

第四节　阴狐疝气者,偏有小大,时时上下,蜘蛛散主之。

蜘蛛散方:蜘蛛十四枚(熬焦),桂枝半两。

上二味,为散,取八分一匕,饮和服,日再服。蜜丸亦可。

4. Zhi-zhu-san (Spider and Cinnamon Formula) shrinks a scrotal hernia that grows large on some occasions and small on others and frequently ascends and descends.

14 pcs. charred spiders　　　　　　　　0.5 liang cinnamon

Pulverize the ingredients. One-eighth of a cubic cun (ca. 0.25g) of the powder mixed with boiled water is taken twice daily. The powder may also be mixed with honey, formed into pills, and taken in that form.

第五节　问曰:病腹痛有虫,其脉何以别之? 师曰:腹中痛,其脉当沉,若弦,反洪大,故有蛔虫。

5. The disciples asked: "How can we tell by the pulse if a patient's abdominal aching is due to worms?"

The master replied: "Abdominal aching usually reflects a submerged pulse but if the pulse feels chordal, and yet surging and big, it signifies worms."

第六节　蛔虫之为病,令人吐涎,心痛,发作有时,毒药不止,甘草粉蜜汤主之。

甘草粉蜜汤方:甘草二两,粉一两,蜜四两。

上三味,以水三升,先煮甘草,取二升,去滓,内粉、蜜,搅令和,煎如薄粥。温服一升,差即止。

6. Worms cause slobbering, heartburn and aching, and seizures at fixed hours that cannot be halted by poisonous drugs. Gan-Cao-fen-mi-tang (Licorice, White Lead, and Hone Combination) is required.

2 liang licorice　　　　　　　　　　4 liang honey

1 liang white lead

First place the licorice in 3 sheng of water and decoct until 2 sheng remains. Discard the dregs and add the other ingredients. Stir as the mixture decocts until it is of a thin congee consistency.

One sheng at a time is taken warmed. Suspend administration when the patient is cured.

第七节　蛔厥者,当吐蛔,令病者静而复时烦,此为脏寒,蛔上入膈,故烦,须臾复止,得食而呕又烦者,就闻食臭出,其人常自吐蛔。

7. A patient with "ascarid faint" vomits the parasites. If the afflicted becomes quiescent and frequently experiences short spells of discomfort, it is due to visceral chills which cause the parasites to ascend into the diaphragm and create the discomfort. Vomiting and irritation after eating occur because the parasites are seeking the food. One so infected will vomit the worms.

第八节　蛔厥者,乌梅丸主之。

乌梅丸方：乌梅三百个,细辛六两(炮),黄连一斤,当归四两,黄柏六两,桂枝六两,人参六两,干姜十两,川椒四两(去汗),附子六两(炮)。

上十味,异捣筛,合治之,以苦酒渍乌梅一宿,去核,蒸之五升米下,饭熟,捣成泥,和药令相得,内臼中,与蜜杵二千下,丸如梧子大,先食饮服十丸,日三服,稍加至二十丸。禁生冷滑臭等食。

8. Wu-mei-wan (Mume Formula) treats "ascarid faint."

300 pcs. mume fruits	6 liang phellodendron
6 liang asarum	6 liang cinnamon
6 liang baked aconite	6 liang ginseng
16 liang coptis	10 liang dried ginger
4 liang danggui	4 liang zanthoxylum with the oil removed

Pound each of the above ingredients except the mume into powder separately and then mix together. Pickle the mume in vinegar overnight, remove the kernels, place under 5 sheng of rice, and steam until the rice is well cooked. Pound the rice and the mume together to form a paste, then add the rest of the ingredients powdered to form an evenly blended mass. Place the mass in a mortar with honey and pound 2 000 times. Make into pills each the size of a sterculia seed. Ten pills are taken before meals three times a day. The dosage should be gradually increased to 20 pills. Cold, slippery, raw, or fetid food is forbidden.

妇人妊娠病脉证并治第二十

XX.

On Pulse Syndrome Complex and
Treatment of Gynopathy during Pregnancy

第一节　师曰：妇人得平脉，阴脉小弱，其人渴，不能食，无寒热，名妊娠，桂枝汤主之。方见下利中。于法六十日，当有此证，设有医治逆者，却一月加吐下者，则绝之。

1. The master said："The pulse of a woman patient is moderate, but the pulse at the Cubit is slender and weak. She is also thirsty and has no appetite. No fever or chill is observed. This indicates a pregnancy, she should take Gui-zhi-tang (Cinnamon Combination). As a rule these symptoms appear during the first sixty days of pregnancy; if the doctor mistreats the conformation as common nausea and causes the woman to develop vomiting and diarrhea for one month, stop all medication and treatment. The patient should recover spontaneously.

第二节　妇人宿有癥病，经断未及三月，而得漏下不止，胎动在脐上者，为癥痼害。妊娠六月动者，前三月经水利时胎也。下血者，后断三月衃也。所以血不止者，其癥不去故也，当下其癥，桂枝茯苓丸主之。

桂枝茯苓丸方：桂枝、茯苓、牡丹（去心）、芍药、桃仁（去皮尖，熬）各等分。

上五味，末之，炼蜜和丸，如兔屎大，每日食前服一丸。不知，加至三丸。

2. Movement above the navel and sudden incessant uterine bleeding three months after cessation of menses indicates the presence of a tumor. However, movement in the sixth month with regular menses in the first three months signals pregnancy. Blood discharged in the first three months is vicious (stagnant) blood, but incessant uterine bleeding is due to a tumor which should be discharged with Gui-zhi-fu-ling-wan (Cinnamon and Hoelen Formula).

cinnamon	cored peony
hoelen	peach seeds with apex and skin removed
equal amounts of each	

Powder the ingredients, knead with honey, and make into pills the size of rabbit pellets. One pill is taken before meals. If no effect occurs, the dosage should be increased to three pills.

第三节　妇人怀娠六七月,脉弦,发热,其胎愈胀,腹痛恶寒者,少腹如扇,所以然者,子脏开故也,当以附子汤温其脏。方未见。

3. If a woman in her sixth or seventh month of pregnancy develops a chordal pulse, a fever, a feeling of increasing distention of the fetus, abdominal aching, chillphobia, and a feeling of cold in the lower abdomen, her womb has an opening. Fu-zi-tang (Aconite Combination) warms the womb. (The contents of Fu-zi-tang are not listed in the original text)

第四节　师曰:妇人有漏下者,有半产后因续下血都不绝者,有妊娠下血者,假令妊娠腹中痛,为胞阻,胶艾汤主之。

胶艾汤方:一方加干姜一两。胡氏治妇人胞动,无干姜。川芎、阿胶、甘草各二两,艾叶、当归各三两,芍药四两,干地黄四两。

上七味,以水五升,清酒三升,合煮取三升,去滓,内胶,令消尽,温服一升,日三服。不差,更作。

4. Jiao-ai-tang (Gelatin and Artemisia Combination) primarily helps stop uterine bleeding, including incessant bleeding following abortion and bleeding during pregnancy. The formula also treats abdominal aching due to fetal obstruction.

2 liang cnidium	3 liang moxa
2 liang gelatin	4 liang peony
2 liang licorice	6 liang dried rehmannia
3 liang danggui	

Decoct all the ingredients except gelatin in 5 sheng of water and 3 sheng of clear wine until 3 sheng remains. Discard the dregs and stir in the gelatin until completely dissolved. One sheng is taken warmed three times a day. If the patient is not cured, repeat the treatment.

第五节　妇人怀娠,腹中疠痛,当归芍药散主之。

当归芍药散方:当归三两,芍药一斤,芎劳半斤一作三两,茯苓四两,泽泻半斤,白术四两。

上六味,杵为散,取方寸匕,酒和,日三服。

5. Dang-gui-shao-yao-san (Dang-gui and Peony Formula) helps a pregnant woman with abdominal cramping pains.

3 liang dang-gui	4 liang hoelen
16 liang peony	8 liang alisma

3 liang cnidium   4 liang atractylodes

Pulverize the ingredients. One fangcunbi of the peonymixed with wine is taken three times daily.

第六节　妊娠,呕吐不止,干姜人参半夏丸主之。

干姜人参半夏丸方：干姜、人参各一两,半夏二两。

上三味,末之,以生姜汁糊为丸,如梧桐子大,饮服十丸,日三服。

6. Gan-jiang-ren-sheng-ban-xia-wan (Ginger, Ginseng, and Pinellia Formula) stops incessant vomiting in a pregnant woman.

1 liang dried ginger   2 liang pinellia

1 liang ginseng

Pulverize the ingredients, mix with fresh ginger juice, and make into pills, each the size of a sterculia seed. Ten pills are taken with water three times a day.

第七节　妊娠,小便难,饮食如故,当归贝母苦参丸主之。

当归贝母苦参丸方：当归、贝母、苦参各四两。

上三味,末之,炼蜜丸如小豆大,饮服三丸,加至十丸。

7. A pregnant woman with difficult urination and a normal appetite needs Dang-gui-bei-mu-ku-sheng-wan (Dang-gui and Fritillaria Formula).

4 liang danggui   4 liang sophora (for dysuria in men add 0.5

4 liang fritillaria   liang of talc)

Pulverize the ingredients, knead with honey, and make into pills the size of a small bean. Three pills at a time are taken with water. Dosage may be increased to ten pills.

第八节　妊娠,有水气,身重,小便不利,洒淅恶寒,起即头眩,葵子茯苓散主之。

葵子茯苓散方：葵子一升,茯苓三两。

上二味,杵为散,饮服方寸匕,日三服,小便利则愈。

8. A pregnant woman with edema, a feeling of generalized heaviness, oliguria, morbid chillphobia, and dizziness on standing primarily requires Gui-zi-fu-ling-san (Abutilon and Hoelen Formula).

1 sheng abutilon   3 liang hoelen

Pound the ingredients into powder. One fangcunbi with water is taken three times a day. Copious urination signals recovery.

第九节　妇人妊娠,宜常服当归散主之。

当归散方：当归、黄芩、芍药、川芎各一斤，白术半斤。

上五味，杵为散，酒饮服方寸匕，日再服，妊娠常服即易产，胎无疾苦，产后百病悉主之。

9. Dang-gui-san (Danggui Formula) taken frequently benefits pregnant women.

16 liang danggui   16 liang peony

16 liang scute   16 liang cnidium

8 liang atractylodes

Pulverize the ingredients. One fangcunbi of the powder is taken with wine twice daily. If a woman takes this formula throughout her pregnancy, she will easily deliver a healthy baby. A woman taking this formula will also be free from all diseases after delivery.

第十节　妊娠养胎，白术散主之。

白术散方：见《外台》。白术四分，川芎四分，蜀椒三分(去汗)，牡蛎二分。

上四味，杵为散；酒服一钱匕，日三服，夜一服。但苦痛，加芍药；心下毒痛，倍加川芎；心烦吐痛，不能食饮，加细辛一两，半夏大者二十枚，服之后，更以醋浆水服之，若呕，以醋浆水服之复不解者，小麦汁服之；已后渴者，大麦粥服之。病虽愈，服之勿置。

10. Bai-shu-san (Atractylodes and Cnidium Formula) nourishes the fetus during pregnancy.

4 fen atractylodes   3 fen zanthoxylum with oil removed

4 fen cnidium   2 fen oyster shell

Pulverize the ingredients. One cubic cun is taken with wine three times during the day and once at night. If the patient has pain only, incorporate peony; if the patient has severe pain beneath the heart, double the amount of cnidium; if the patient has annoyance in the heart, vomits with aching, and cannot eat, add one tael of asarum and 20 corms of large pinellia. If after taking the formula, the patient vomits, give her vinegar. If it does not work, give wheat juice to relieve vomiting. For thirst after the above symptoms are gone, give barley congee. The formula should be taken continuously even after recovery.

第十一节　妇人伤胎，怀身腹满，不得小便，从腰以下，重如有水气状，怀身七月，太阴当养不养，此心气实，当刺泻劳宫及关元，小便微利则愈。

11. In the seventh month of pregnancy the greater yin meridian nourishes the fetus. If firmness of heart Qi occurs as a consequence of contraction of a shang hah disease, an exuberant heart and intestinal fire will injure the greater yin meridian, which in turn causes injury of the fetus. The symptoms of abdominal distention, oliguria, and heaviness with an edematous appearance below the waist should be purged by puncturing the lao gong and guan yuan points in order to slightly increase urination and bring about recovery.

妇人产后病脉证治第二十一

XXI.

On Pulse Syndrome Complex and
Treatment of Postpartum Diseases

第一节 问曰:新产妇人有三病,一者病痉,二者病郁冒,三者大便难,何谓也?

师曰:新产血虚,多汗出,喜中风,故令病痉;亡血复汗,寒多,故令郁冒;亡津液胃燥,故令大便难。

1. The disciples asked: "Why do postpartum women commonly suffer from convulsions, dizziness, and difficulty in defecation?"

The master replied: "Immediately after labor a woman suffers from blood weakness and perspires profusely, making her susceptible to the wind and hence convulsions. The loss of blood along with perspiration and chills causes depressive dizziness whereas the depletion of body fluids leads to stomach aridity and hence makes defecating difficult."

第二节 产妇郁冒,其脉微弱,呕不能食,大便反坚,但头汗出。所以然者,血虚而厥,厥而必冒。冒家欲解,必大汗出,以血虚下厥,孤阳上出,故头汗出。所以产妇喜汗出者,亡阴血虚,阳气独盛,故当汗出,阴阳乃复。大便坚,呕不能食,小柴胡汤主之。

2. When a puerperal woman has depressive dizziness and a minute and weak pulse, vomits and has no appetite, passes hard stools, and perspires on the head only, it is due to blood weakness and its consequent flushing of yang. The flushing definitely results in dizziness and the patient perspires profusely before the dizziness is relieved. Blood weakness and chills in the lower warmer lead to flushing of solitary yang and consequently sweating on the head. A puerperal woman needs to perspire because exhaustion of yin and blood weakness lead to excessive yang. Sweating restores the balance of yin and yang. Xiao-chai-hu-tang (Minor Bupleurum Combination) treats a conformation of hard stools, vomiting, and loss of appetite.

第三节　病解能食,七八日更发热者,此为胃实,大承气汤主之。

3．If the woman regains her appetite after taking Minor Bupleurum Combination but has a relapse of a fever seven or eight days later, she has gastric firmness and primarily needs Da-cheng-qi-tang (Major Rhubarb Combination).

第四节　产后腹中疙痛,当归生姜羊肉汤主之;并治腹中寒疝,虚劳不足。

4．Dang-gui-sheng-jiang-yang-rou-tang (Danggui, Ginger, and Mutton Combination) treats puerperal abdominal cramping pain, chill colic in the abdomen, and other symptoms derived from weakness, fatigue, and deficiency.

第五节　产后腹痛,烦满不得卧,枳实芍药散主之。
枳实芍药散方: 枳实(烧令黑,勿太过)、芍药等分。
上二味,杵为散,服方寸匕,日三服,并主痈脓,以麦粥下之。

5．Zhi-shi-shao-yao-san (Zhi shi and Peony Formula) treats postpartum abdominal aching with distress and abdominal distention that renders the afflicted unable to lie down.

Zhi-shi burnt black but not over burnt　　　　peony

equal amounts of each

Pulverize the ingredients. One fangcunbi is taken three times a day. This formula also treats carbuncular pustulation; in such cases it is taken with barley congee.

第六节　师曰:产妇腹痛,法当以枳实芍药散,假令不愈者,此为腹中有干血着脐下,宜下瘀血汤主之;亦主经水不利。
下瘀血汤方: 大黄三两,桃仁二十枚,蟅虫二十枚(熬,去足)。
上三味,末之,炼蜜和为四丸,以酒杯一升,煎一丸,取八合顿服之,新血下如豚肝。

6．The master said: "As a rule Zhi shi and Peony Formula relieves postpartum abdominal aching. However, if the formula is ineffective, it is due to the presence of dry blood lodged in the abdomen beneath the navel. This condition requires Xia-yu-xue-tang (Persica and Eupolyphaga Combination), a formula which also treats scanty menstruation."

3 liang rhubarb　　　　　　　　　　20 pcs. roasted eupolyphaga

20 pcs. persica kernels (Eupolyphaga　　　with the legs removed

sinensis)

Pulverize the ingredients, knead with honey, and make into four balls. Decoct one ball in one sheng of wine until 0.8 sheng remains. The decoction is taken in one draft. Fresh blood clots resembling pig liver will be discharged.

第七节　产后七八日,无太阳证,少腹坚痛,此恶露不尽,不大便,烦躁发热,切脉微实,再倍发热,日晡时烦躁者,本食,食则谵语,至夜即愈,宜大承气汤主之。热在里,结在膀胱也。

7. If a woman develops hardening and aching in the lower abdomen but no greater yang symptoms seven or eight days after labor, she has not completely discharged the lochia. However, a minute and full pulse, constipation, discomfort and irritation with fever and no appetite, the discomfort, irritation, and fever becoming more severe toward dusk and delirium occurring after eating but disappearing at night signals that a fever has stagnated in the interior and is bound in the urinary bladder. Such a woman requires Da-cheng-qi-tang (Major Rhubarb Combination).

第八节　产后风,续之数十日不解,头微痛,恶寒,时时有热,心下闷,干呕,汗出,虽久,阳旦证续在耳,可与阳旦汤。

8. A patient who has been suffering from evil wind without relief for twenty to thirty days after delivery-mild headache, chillphobia, frequent fever, depression beneath the heart, dry heaves, and excessive perspiration has a Gui-zhi-tang(Cinnamon Combination) conformation. Despite the length of suffering, this formula may be given.

第九节　产后中风,发热,面正赤,喘而头痛,竹叶汤主之。
竹叶汤方：竹叶一把,葛根三两,防风、桔梗、桂枝、人参、甘草各一两,附子一枚(炮),大枣十五枚,生姜五两。
上十味,以水一斗,煮取二升半,分温三服,温覆使汗出。颈项强,用大附子一枚,破之如豆大,煎药扬去沫。呕者,加半夏半升洗。

9. A puerperal woman with "contraction of winds" fever reflected in a ruddy facial complexion, gasping, and headache needs Zhu-ye-tang (Bamboo Leaves Combination).

1 handful bamboo leaves	1 liang ginseng
3 liang pueraria	1 liang licorice
1 liang siler	1 pc. baked aconite root
1 liang platycodon	15 pcs. jujube fruits
1 liang cinnamon	5 liang fresh ginger

Decoct the ingredients in 10 sheng of water until 2.5 sheng remains. Divide the decoction into three portions. One portion is taken at a time. Keep the patient warm by wrapping her in quilts to induce perspiration. If the patient develops stiffness in the neck, break a large aconite root into pieces the size of beans and decoct. Remove the foam and give the decoction to the patient. If the patient vomits, add 0.5 sheng of washed pinellia.

第十节　妇人乳中虚,烦乱呕逆,安中益气,竹皮大丸主之。

竹皮大丸方：生竹茹二分,石膏二分,桂枝一分,甘草七分,白薇一分。

上五味,末之,枣肉和丸弹子大,以饮服一丸,日三夜一服。有热者,倍白薇,烦喘者,加柏实一分。

10. During puerperal time a woman with a feeling of weakness, discomfort, derangement, and regurgitation needs Zhu-pi-da-wan (Gypsum and Bamboo Formula) to settle her stomach and enrich her vitality.

2 fen raw bamboo taenia　　　　　　　　　7 fen licorice

2 fen gypsum　　　　　　　　　　　　　　1 fen cynanchum

1 fen cinnamon

Pulverize the ingredients, mix with jujube flesh, and make into pills the size of a bullet. One pill is taken with water three times a day and twice a night. If the patient has a fever, double the amount of cynanchum; if the patient has discomfort and asthma, add one fen of biota fruit.

第十一节　产后下利虚极,白头翁加甘草阿胶汤主之。

白头翁加甘草阿胶汤方：白头翁、甘草、阿胶各二两,秦皮、黄连、柏皮各三两。

上六味,以水七升,煮取二升半,内胶令消尽,分温三服。

11. Bai-tou-weng-jia-gan-cao-e-jiao-tang (Anemone, Licorice, and Gelatin Combination) treats postpartum diarrhea and extreme weakness.

2 liang anemone　　　　　　　　　　　3 liang fraxinus

2 liang licorice　　　　　　　　　　　　3 liang coptis

2 liang gelatin　　　　　　　　　　　　3 liang phellodendron

Decoct all the ingredients except the gelatin in 7 sheng of water until 2.5 sheng remains. Add the gelatin and after it dissolves completely, divide the decoction into three portions. Each portion is taken warmed.

附方1：

《千金》三物黄芩汤：治妇人在草蓐,自发露得风,四肢苦烦热,头痛者与小柴胡汤;头不痛但烦者,此汤主之。黄芩一两,苦参二两,干地黄四两。

上三味,以水八升,煮取二升,温服一升,多吐下虫。

Two other formulas are also frequently given to puerperal women. When a puerperal woman has contracted wind evil because of exposure of her lower body during labor and thus has limb distress, annoying fever, and a headache, she can be given Xiao-chai-hu-tang (Minor Bupleurum Combination); if she has only annoyance and no headache, she should be treated with San-wu-huang-qin-tang (Scute Three Herb Combination).

1 liang scute   4 liang dried rehmannia

2 liang sophora

Decoct the ingredients in 6 sheng of water until 2 sheng remains. One sheng is taken warmed. The drug causes the patient to vomit or discharge a large number of worms.

附方2：

《千金》内补当归建中汤：治妇人产后虚羸不足，腹中刺痛不止，吸吸少气，或苦少腹中急，摩痛引腰背，不能食饮，产后一月，日得服四、五剂为善，令人强壮，宜。

当归四两，桂枝三两，芍药六两，生姜三两，甘草二两，大枣十二枚。

上六味，以水一斗，煮取三升，分温三服，一日令尽。若大虚，加饴糖六两，汤成内之，于火上煖，令饴消。若去血过多，崩伤内衄不止，加地黄六两，阿胶二两，合八味，汤成内阿胶。若无当归，以芎䓖代之。若无生姜，以干姜代之。

Postpartum feebleness and deficiency, incessant stabbing pains in the abdomen, difficult breathing, urgency in the lower abdomen with cramping pains extending to the lower back, and inability to eat and drink requires Nei-bu-dang-gui-jian-zhong-tang (Dang-gui, Cinnamon, and Peony Combination). It is recommended that for the best effects women should take four to five doses of this formula every day for one month after delivery. It strengthens.

4 liang dang-gui   3 liang fresh ginger

3 liang cinnamon   2 liang licorice

6 liang peony   12 pcs. jujubes

Decoct the herbs in 10 sheng of water until 3 sheng remains. Divide into three portions. One portion at a time is taken warmed. The entire decoction should be drunk within one day. If the patient is very weak, add 6 taels of maltose to the decoction and warm on a fire to dissolve. If the patient has lost a lot of blood from uterine bleeding or internal bleeding, add 6 taels of rehmannia and 2 taels of gelatin. The gelatin is added after the other herbs have been decocted. If dang-gui is not available, use cnidium in its place. If fresh ginger is unavailable, use dried ginger.

妇人杂病脉证并治第二十二

XXII.

On Pulse Syndrome Complex and
Treatment of Miscellaneous Gynecological Diseases

第一节　妇人中风七八日,续来寒热,发作有时,经水适断,此为热入血室,其血必结,故使如疟状,发作有时,小柴胡汤主之。

1. A woman with "contraction of winds" has alternating seizures of chills and fever at fixed hours. The seizures last for seven to eight days and interrupt the menses. The fever invading the womb causes the blood to stagnate and produces malarialtype symptoms. The woman requires treatment with Xiao-chai-hu-tang (Minor Bupleurum Combination).

第二节　妇人伤寒发热,经水适来,昼日明了,暮则谵语,如见鬼状者,此为热入血室,治之无犯胃气及上二焦,必自愈。

2. A fever has invaded the womb of a woman who in the beginning of her menses suffers from shang han (severe chills and fever). At dusk she will be delirious acting, as though she has met a ghost, but will feel good in the daytime. An appropriate exsanguinative that won't upset gastric Qi or affect the upper and middle warmers will cure the disease.

第三节　妇人中风,发热恶寒,经水适来,得之七八日,热除脉迟,身凉和,胸胁满,如结胸状,谵语者,此为热入血室也,当刺期门,随其实而取之。

3. Sometimes a woman contracts evil wind with fever and chillphobia at the onset of menses. If seven to eight days later the fever subsides, the pulse slows, and the body cools, but the chest and ribs feel taut and delirium has set in, a fever has invaded the womb. The firm fever should be purged by acupuncture applied at the qimen point. Extent of treatment depends on the degree of firmness of the fever.

第四节　阳明病,下血谵语者,此为热入血室,但头汗出,当刺期门,随其实而泻之,濈然汗出则愈。

4. A fever has invaded the womb of a woman who is delirious, has sunlight yang disease, and discharges blood. If she perspires on the head only, it is necessary to purge the firm fire by inserting acupuncture needles on the qimen point until she perspires all over her body; thereby the condition is relieved.

第五节　妇人咽中如有炙脔,半夏厚朴汤主之。
半夏厚朴汤方:半夏一升,厚朴三两,茯苓四两,生姜五两,干苏叶二两。
上五味,以水七升,煮取四升,分温四服,日三夜一服。

5. A woman who feels as if a piece of broiled meat is stuck in her throat should take Ban-xia-hou-pu-tang (Pinellia and Magnolia Combination).

1 sheng pinellia	5 liang fresh ginger
3 liang magnolia bark	2 liang dry perilla leaves
4 liang hoelen	

Decoct the herbs in 7 sheng of water until 4 sheng remains, then divide the decoction into four portions. One portion warmed is taken three times a day and once at night.

第六节　妇人脏躁,喜悲伤欲哭,象如神灵所作,数欠伸,甘麦大枣汤主之。
甘麦大枣汤方:甘草三两,小麦一升,大枣十枚。
上三味,以水六升,煮取三升,温分三服。亦补脾气。

6. A woman with visceral irritation (hysteria) tends to grieve and cry as though possessed by a spirit. She also yawns frequently. She needs Gan-mai-da-zao-tang (Licorice and Jujube Combination).

3 liang licorice	10 pcs. jujubes
1 sheng wheat	

Decoct the herbs with 6 sheng of water until 3 sheng remains, then divide the decoction into three portions. Each portion is taken warmed. This formula supplements splenic Qi.

第七节　妇人吐涎沫,医反下之,心下即痞,当先治其吐涎沫,小青龙汤主之;涎沫止,乃治痞,泻心汤主之。

7. A slobbering woman who undergoes purgation only to have a resulting obstruction beneath

the heart should first be given Xiao-qing-long-tang (Minor Blue Dragon Combination) to arrest the slobbering. After the slobbering has ceased, Xie-xin-tang (Coptis and Rhubarb Combination) will relieve the obstruction.

第八节　妇人之病,因虚、积冷、结气,为诸经水断绝,至有历年,血寒积结胞门,寒伤经络,凝坚在上,呕吐涎唾,久成肺痈,形体损分;在中盘结,绕脐寒疝;或两胁疼痛,与脏相连;或结热中,痛在关元,脉数无疮,肌若鱼鳞,时着男子,非止女身。在下未多,经候不匀。令阴掣痛,少腹恶寒;或引腰脊,下根气街,气冲急痛,膝胫疼烦,奄忽眩冒,状如厥癫;或有忧惨,悲伤多嗔,此皆带下,非有鬼神,久则羸瘦,脉虚多寒。三十六病,千变万端,审脉阴阳,虚实紧弦,行其针药,治危得安,其虽同病,脉各异源,子当辨记,勿谓不然。

8. Many gynecological problems result from weakness, stale chills, and "jie Qi." Women so afflicted may have suppressed menstruation lasting for years; cold blood accumulating and binding in the womb; and chills that injure and cause coagulation and hardening of the meridians. If the condition occurs in the upper warmer, vomiting and slobbering and eventually development of pulmonary carbuncles result in emaciation of the body. If the condition is confined to the middle warmer, there will be chill colic around the navel, or pain in the ribs and involvement of the viscera, or fever confined to the interior manifesting aching at the Guanyuan area (3 inches beneath the navel), a quick pulse, and no sores but coarse skin resembling fish scales. The condition often afflicts males, too. Exhaustion of the belt meridian, not spirits or ghosts, causes scanty or copious menstruation; abnormal menstruation; dragging pain at the genitalia; chill phobia in the lower abdomen involving the waist and spine and extending down to the Qijie point; acute pain of Qi flushing; aching and discomfort in the knees and calves; dizziness and vertigo resembling fainting and madness; or bouts of sorrow, misery, grief, and anger. If the symptoms, persist the patient becomes emaciated and develops an empty pulse and chills. The thirty-six diseases that derive from the exhaustion of the belt meridian have countless variations. Hence, it is mandatory to carefully discriminate between yin and yang, emptiness and forcefulness, and tenseness and chordalness, before applying acupuncture and herbal treatments to secure and save patients who may have the same disease but may have different pulses reflecting different etiologies. This rule must be remembered and not be regarded with indifference.

第九节　问曰:妇人年五十所,病下利,数十日不止,暮即发热,少腹里急,腹满,手掌烦热。唇口干燥,何也?

师曰:此病属带下。何以故? 曾经半产,瘀血在少腹不去。何以知之? 其证唇口干燥,故知之。当以温经汤主之。

温经汤方:吴茱萸三两,当归、芎劳、芍药、人参、桂枝、阿胶、牡丹皮(去心)、生姜、甘草各二两,半夏半升,麦门冬一升(去心)。

上十二味,以水一斗,煮取三升,分温三服;亦主妇人少腹寒,久不受胎;兼取崩中去血,或月水来过多,及至期不来。

9. The disciples asked: "Why would a woman of about fifty who had discharge of blood for twenty to thirty days develop a fever at dusk, an urgent sensation in the lower abdomen, a full abdomen, an annoying fever in the palms, and dry lips?"

The master answered: "This is one of the diseases of exhaustion of the belt meridian. She has aborted and the extravasated blood has stagnated in the lower abdomen. How do we know this? Her dry lips tell the story." Treatment calls primarily for Wen-jing-tang (Dang-gui and Evodia Combination).

3 liang evodia	2 liang gelatin
2 liang dang-gui	2 liang cored moutan
2 liang cnidium	2 liang fresh ginger
2 liang peony	2 liang licorice
2 liang ginseng	0.5 sheng pinellia
2 liang cinnamon	1 sheng cored ophiopogon

Place the ingredients in 10 sheng of water and decoct until 3 sheng remains. Divide the decoction into three portions. Each portion is taken warmed. This formula aids women with chills in the lower abdomen and long term infecundity; metrorrhagia with loss of blood; or excessive or scanty menses.

第十节　带下经水不利,少腹满痛,经一月再见者,土瓜根散主之。
土瓜根散方:土瓜根、芍药、桂枝、䗪虫各三两。
上四味,杵为散,酒服方寸匕,日三服。

10. Women with "exhaustion of the belt meridian" resulting in scanty menses, distention and aching of the lower abdomen, and menstrual periods twice monthly should primarily take Tu-gua-gen-san (Cucumeroides Formula).

3 liang thladiantha tuba	3 liang peony
3 liang cinnamon	3 liang eupolyphaga

Pound the ingredients into powder. One fangcunbi of the powder is taken with wine three times a day.

第十一节　寸口脉弦而大,弦则为减,大则为芤,减则为寒,芤则为虚,虚寒相搏,此名曰革,妇人则半产漏下,旋覆花汤主之。

11. A chordal and big pulse on the cun site is significant in that the chordal characteristic in-

dicates reduction resulting in chills and the bigness, hollowness or emptiness. An interaction between chills and emptiness leads to a tympanic pulse, the same pulse observed in abortions or uterine bleeding. Treatment requires Xuan-fu-hua-tang (Inula Combination).

第十二节　妇人陷经,漏下,黑不解,胶姜汤主之。

12. A woman suffering from continuous menstruation of black blood needs Jiao-Jiang-tang (Gelatin and Ginger Combination).

第十三节　妇人少腹满如敦状,小便微难而不渴,生后者,此为水与血俱结在血室也,大黄甘遂汤主之。
大黄甘遂汤方:大黄四两,甘遂二两,阿胶二两。
上三味,以水三升,煮取一升,顿服之,其血当下。

13. A woman with a swollen lower abdomen that looks like a dune, slight dysuria, and no thirst following delivery has stagnated water and blood in the womb. She should take Da-huang-gan-sui-tang (Rhubarb, Gansui, and Gelatin Combination).

4 liang rhubarb　　　　　　　　　2 liang gelatin

2 liang gan-sui

Decoct the ingredients in 3 sheng of water until one sheng remains. The decoction is taken in one draft to discharge the stagnated blood.

第十四节　妇人经水不利下,抵当汤主之;亦男子膀胱满急治有瘀血者。
抵当汤方:水蛭三十个(熬),虻虫三十枚(熬,去翅足),桃仁二十个(去皮尖),大黄三两(酒浸)。
上四味,为末,以水五升,煮取三升,去滓,温服一升。

14. A woman with scanty menses should take Di-dang-tang (Rhubarb and Leech Combination). (This formula also treats men's urinary bladder distention and urgency due to stagnated blood)

30 pcs. baked leeches　　　　　　　3 liang wine-pickled rhubarb

30 pcs. baked tabanus (gadflies) with　20 pcs. persica seeds with apex and skin removed
wings and legs removed

Pulverize the ingredients and decoct in 5 sheng of water until 3 sheng remains. Discard the dregs. One sheng is taken warmed.

第十五节　妇人经水闭不利,脏坚癖不止,中有干血,下白物,矾石丸主之。

矾石丸方：矾石三分(烧)，杏仁一分。
上二味，末之，炼蜜和丸枣核大，内脏中，剧者再内之。

15. A woman with suppressed menstruation, continuous formation of hard masses containing dry blood in the womb, and a whitish discharge needs Fan-shi-wan (Alum Formula).

3 fen burnt alum   1 fen apricot seed

Pulverize the ingredients, mix with honey, and make into pills each the size of a jujube kernel. One pill is inserted into the vagina; for a severe condition two pills in succession are used.

第十六节　妇人六十二种风，及腹中血气刺痛，红蓝花酒主之。
红蓝花酒方：红蓝花一两。
上一味，以酒一大升，煎减半，顿服一半，未止，再服。

16. Hong-lan-hua-jiu (Carthamus and Wine Formula) treats the stabbing pain resulting from Qi and blood in the abdomen. The symptom accompanies sixty-two different women's wind diseases.

1 liang carthamus

Place the herb in one big sheng of wine and decoct until the volume has been reduced by half. Half of the decoction is taken. If the pain does not cease, the other half should be used.

第十七节　妇人腹中诸疾痛，当归芍药散主之。

17. Dang-gui-shao-yao-san (Danggui and Peony Formula) treats various women's abdominal problems.

第十八节　妇人腹中痛，小建中汤主之。

18. A woman with abdominal aching should take Xiao-jian-zhong-tang (Minor Cinnamon and Peony Combination).

第十九节　问曰：妇人病，饮食如故，烦热不得卧，而反倚息者，何也？
师曰：此名转胞不得溺也，以胞系了戾，故致此病，但利小便则愈，宜肾气丸主之。

19. The disciples asked: "Why would a woman with a normal appetite suffer from an annoying fever whereby she cannot lie down flat but must rest upright in order to breathe?"

The master said: "The condition is known as 'shift of the bladder' and it makes the patient incapable of urinating. Tangled ureters cause the problem; it can be relieved by rendering urination with Ba-wei-di-huang-wan (Rehmannia Eight Formula)."

第二十节　妇人阴寒,温阴中坐药,蛇床子散主之。
蛇床子散方:蛇床子仁。
上一味,末之,以白粉少许,和令相得,如枣大,绵裹内之,自然温。

20. A woman with genital chills needs to have the interior of the vagina warmed with She-chuang-zi-san (Selinum Formula):

Selinum, white lead powder

Pulverize the selinum and mix evenly with enough white lead powder to make a mass as large as a jujube fruit. Wrap in silk and insert into the vagina. This warms the vagina.

第二十一节　少阴脉滑而数者,阴中即生疮,阴中蚀疮烂者,狼牙汤洗之。
狼牙汤方:狼牙三两。
上一味,以水四升,煮取半升,以缠筋如茧,浸汤沥阴中,日四遍。

21. A lesser yin pulse that is slippery and quick signifies sores and ulcers in the vagina. Treatment requires washing of the vagina with Lang-ya-tang (Potentilla Combination).

3 liang potentilla

Place the herb in 4 sheng of water and decoct until the volume is reduced by half. Soak a piece of silk that is tied and bound, resembling the form of a silkworm cocoon, in the decoction. Insertion of the saturated silk into the vagina cleanses it. The cleansing should be done four times a day.

第二十二节　胃气下泄,阴吹而正喧,此谷气之实也,膏发煎导之。
猪膏半斤,乱发如鸡子大三枚。
上二味,和膏中煎之,发消药成,分再服。

22. Gao-fa-jian (Lard and Human Hair Combination) treats downward discharge of gastric Qi that results in breaking wind with a continuous loud sound in the vagina. The condition results from firmness of gu Qi. This formula guides gu Qi out through the rectum.

8 liang lard　　　　　　　　　　　　3 balls human hair (each ball the size of an egg)

Decoct both ingredients until the hair is dissolved completely. Divide the dicoction into two portions. One portionis taken twice a day.

杂疗方第二十三

XXIII.

Miscellaneous Remedies

第一节　退五脏虚热，四时加减柴胡饮子方。

冬三月加柴胡八分，白术八分，陈皮五分，大腹槟榔四枚，(并皮子用)生姜五分，桔梗七分。

春三月加枳实，减白术共六味。

夏三月加生姜三分，枳实五分，甘草三分。共八味

秋三月加陈皮三分，共六味上各㕮咀，分为三贴，一贴以水三升，煮取二升，分温三服，如人行四五里，进一服。如四体壅，添甘草少许，每贴分作三小贴，每小贴以水一升，煮取七合，温服，再合滓为一服，重煮，都成四服。

1. In accordance with the four seasons, Modified Chai-hu-yin-zi (Bupleurum and Areca Combination) relieves weakness and fever of the five viscera.

In the winter use:

8 fen bupleurum	5 fen citrus
8 fen atractylodes	5 fen fresh ginger
4 areca nuts including pericarp and seeds	7 fen platycodon

In the spring substitute zhishi for the atractylodes.

In the summer add:

3 fen fresh ginger	3 fen licorice
5 fen zhi shi	

And in the autumn add 3 fen more of citrus.

Divide the ingredients into three portions and shred them. Decoct each portion in 3 sheng of water until 2 sheng remains. The decoction is divided into three portions and a portion is taken warmed at intervals as long as it takes to walk four to five lis. If he has a heavy feeling, then add a little licorice to each dose, divide each dose into three subdoses, and decoct each subdose with one sheng of water until 0.7 sheng remains. The solution is taken warmed. The dregs of the three subdoses are then combined and decocted again, making a fourth dose.

第二节　长服诃梨勒丸方：诃梨勒,陈皮,厚朴各三两。
上三味,末之,炼蜜丸如梧子大,酒饮服二十丸,加至三十丸。

2．Ke-li-le-wan (Terminalia Formula) is for long term use.

3 liang terminalia　　　　　　　　　　3 liang magnolia bark

3 liang citrus

Pulverize the ingredients, knead with honey, and form into pills the size of a sterculia seed. Each time twenty, increasing to thirty, pills are taken with wine.

第三节　三物备急丸方：大黄一两,干姜一两,巴豆一两(去皮心,熬,外研如脂)。
上药各须精新,先捣大黄、干姜为末,研巴豆内中,合治一千杵,用为散,蜜和丸亦佳,密器中贮之,莫令歇。主心腹诸卒暴百病,若中恶客忤,心腹胀满,卒痛如锥刺,气急口噤,停尸卒死者,以暖水若酒,服大豆许三四丸,或不下,捧头起,灌令下咽,须臾当差。如未差,更与三丸,当腹中鸣,即吐下便差。若口噤,亦须折齿灌之。

3．San-wu-bei-ji-wan (Rhubarb, Ginger, and Croton Formula), a fairly effective medication for emergency use, comes from *Qian Jin Fang*.

1 liang rhubarb　　　　　　　　　　1 liang croton seeds

1 liang dried ginger

After removing the seed coat from the croton, stew it, and then separately grind into a thick paste. Pound the rhubarb and dried ginger into a powder, blend in the croton, and pound one thousand times. Use as a powder or blend with honey and make into pills. Once prepared, the drug should be stored in an airtight container. The formula treats various acute seizures of the heart and abdomen; sudden arrested breathing; infantile neurosis; a distended feeling in the heart and abdomen; sudden stinging pain; shortness of breath with a closed mouth; fainting; and sudden impending death. Three or four pills the size of a soya bean are taken with warm water and vinegar. If the patient is too weak to take the drug, raise his head and pour the mixture down his throat; he should respond immediately. If he does not, give him three more pills. The patient will have borborygmus, vomiting, and diarrhea before recovery. If the patient's mouth will not open, the teeth must be broken.

第四节　治伤寒令愈不复紫石寒食散方：紫石英、白石英、赤石脂、钟乳(碓炼)、栝蒌根、防风、桔梗、文蛤、鬼臼各十分,太一余粮十分(烧),干姜、附子(炮,去皮)、桂枝(去皮)各四分。
上十三味,杵为散,酒服方寸匕。

4. Zi-shi-han-shi-san (Fluorite and Kaolin Formula) treats the shang han condition so that it does not recur.

Fluorite
Quartz ⎫ 10 parts each
Kaolin ⎭

Stalactites (refined with a pestle and mortar)
Trichosanthes
Siler
Platycodon ⎫ 10 parts each
Clams
Diphylleia
Burnt brown hematite

Dried ginger
Roasted and skinned aconite ⎫ 4 parts each
Cinnamon with the coarse outer skin removed

Pound the components into a powder. One cubic cun of the powder is taken with wine.

第五节　救卒死方：薤捣汁灌鼻中。又方：雄鸡冠割取血，管吹内鼻中。猪脂如鸡子大，苦酒一升煮沸灌喉中。鸡肝及血涂面上，以灰围四旁，立起。大豆二十七粒，以鸡子白并酒和，尽以吞之。

5. The following emergency treatments stave off impending death. Pound baker's garlic (Allium bakeri) into juice. Pour the juice into the nostrils.

Spray the blood from a cock's crown into the nose.

Boil a mass of lard as large as an egg with one sheng of vinegar and pour down the patient's throat.

Spread chicken liver and blood on the dying one's face and surround the patient with ashes. (The patient will awaken and rise immediately)

Blend together 27 soya beans, egg white, and wine. Help the patient drink all of it.

第六节　救卒死而目热者方：矾石半斤，以水一斗半煮消，以渍脚令没踝。

6. A formula for a patient with a strong fever who is facing sudden impending death is 8 taels alum boiled in 15 sheng of water until the alum is completely dissolved. Immerse the patient's feet to the ankles in the solution.

第七节　救卒死而目闭者方：骑牛临面,捣薤汁灌耳中,吹皂荚末鼻中,立效。

7. To save a patient whose eyes have closed due to impending death, put the afflicted one face down on an ox; then pour juice from baker's garlic into his ears and spray gleditshchia powder into his nose. The patient will awaken immediately.

第八节　救卒死而张口反折者方：炙手足两爪后十四壮了,饮以五毒诸膏散。

8. For a dying patient whose mouth is open and whose body is bent backward, apply moxibustion to the points behind the finger and toe nails at a rate of 14 units. Then have the patient drink Wu-du-zhu-gao-san with croton.

第九节　救卒死而四肢不收失便者方：马屎一升,水三斗,煮取二斗,以洗之;又取牛洞稀粪也一升温酒灌口中,炙心下一寸,脐上三寸、脐下四寸各一百壮,差。

9. A formula for treating a patient with flaccid limbs and incontinence of urine and feces who is facing sudden impending death is one sheng horse urine boiled in 30 sheng water until 20 sheng remains. The patient is washed with the solution. Analternate formula is one sheng of thin ox excreta boiled with wine and poured into the patient's mouth. One hundred units of moxibustion may be applied to each of the following points: 1 inch beneath the heart, 3 inches above the navel, and 4 inches beneath the navel. The patient will soon recover.

第十节　救小儿卒死而吐利不知是何病方：狗屎一丸,绞取汁以灌之。无湿者,水煮干者取汁。

10. To save a dying child who is vomiting and has diarrhea of an undetermined origin, pour the juice from one ball of moist dog feces into the patient's mouth. If no moist dog feces are available, boil dry ones in water and strain to get the juice.

第十一节　治尸蹶方：尸蹶脉动而无气,气闭不通,故静而死也,治方。菖蒲屑,内鼻两孔中吹之,令人以桂屑着舌下。又方：剔取左角发方寸烧末,酒和,灌令入喉,立起。

11. Two formulas help an unconscious patient whose heart is beating but who is not breathing because the air passage is obstructed. He will appear to be dead. Blow shredded acorus dust in to both nostrils and place cinnamon dust underneath the tongue.

Another life-saving formula is one square inch of hair from the patient's left temple burned to ashes and then blended with wine and poured down the patient's throat. The person will revive at once.

第十二节　救卒死,客忤死,还魂汤主之方：麻黄三两,杏仁七十个,甘草一两(炙)。
上三味,以水八升,煮取三升,去滓,分令咽之,通治诸感忤。

12. Huan-hun-tang (Mahuang, Apricot Seed, and Licorice Combination) saves a patient from sudden impending death or helps a child with infantile neurosis.

3 liang denoded mahuang　　　　　1 liang baked licorice

70 pcs. apricot seeds with seed coats and apexes removed

Boil the three components with 8 sheng of water until 3 sheng remains; strain and discard the dregs. Divide into portions and give to the patient. This formula solves various problems from sudden attacks.

第十三节　又方：
韭根一把,乌梅二十七个,吴茱萸半升(炒)。
上三味,以水一斗煮之,以病人栉内中,三沸,栉浮者生;沉者死。煮取三升,去滓分饮之。

13. Another formula for the dying is this:

1 handful of leek root　　　　　　0.5 sheng fried evodia
27 mume fruits

Place one handful of leek root, 27 mume fruits, and 0.5 sheng fried evodia in 10 sheng of water and decoct. Then place the patient's comb in the decoction and boil for a while longer. If the comb floats, the patient will recover; if the comb sinks, his condition is incurable. (In ancient China, people wore the same comb, made from cowhorn, in their hair for a lifetime. An individual's comb thus would become saturated with his own body oils.) Nevertheless, continuously boil the decoction until three sheng remains. Discard the dregs. The decoction is divided into equal portions and drunk.

第十四节　救自缢死方：救自缢死,旦至暮,虽已冷,必可治;暮至旦,小难也。恐此当言阴气盛故也。然夏时夜短于昼,又热,犹应可治。又云:心下若微温者,一日以上,犹可治之。方:徐徐抱解,不得截绳,上下安被卧之。一人以脚踏其两肩,手少挽其发,常弦弦勿纵之。一人以手按据胸上,数动之;一人摩捋臂胫屈伸之,若已僵,但渐渐强屈之,并按其腹。如此一炊顷,气从口出,呼吸眼开而犹引按莫置,亦勿苦劳之。须臾,可少桂汤及粥清含与之,令濡喉,渐渐能咽,乃稍止。若向令两人以管吹其两耳,扠好。此法最善,无不活者。

14. When a person has hanged himself, he can be revived even though his body has become

cool if the hanging took place between morning and evening. But if the hanging has occurred between evening and the next morning, resuscitation will be a little more difficult. If the patient has quarrelled before hanging himself, his Qi will be exuberant and the conditions favorable to reviving him. In summer the patient is more easily revived because of the long days and hot climate. Also if the area beneath the heart is still warm, the victim can be resuscitated even though the hanging occurred more than one day previously.

To revive the victim, first embrace him; then instead of cutting the rope slowly untie it. Lay him down on quilts and have someone tramp on his shoulders with his feet while you hold his hair with your hands in such a way that the head is always kept taut. Meanwhile another person should massage his chest with quick motions while another one is flexing and extending his arms and legs and massaging his abdomen. The treatment should be continued for about the time of one meal. The victim will exhale air from his mouth and begin to breathe with closed eyes. The healer must continue the massage and extending and flexing maneuvers without interruption. He must not become agonized or fatigued. A while later, Shao-gui-tang and thin rice congee may be given to moisten the victim's throat. Gradually he will become able to swallow. Finally have two persons blow in each ear with a tube. Most victims will respond and awaken.

第十五节　疗中暍方：凡中暍死，不可使得冷，得冷便死，疗之方：屈草带，绕暍人脐，使三两人溺其中，令温。亦可用热泥和屈草，亦可扣瓦椀底，按及车缸，以着耙人，取令溺，须得流去，此谓道路穷，卒无汤，当令溺其中，欲使多人溺，取令温。若有汤便可与之，不可泥及车缸，恐此物冷，暍既在夏月，得热泥土，暖车缸，亦可用也。

15. A sunstruck patient who is close to death should not be subjected to cold, otherwise he will die. He can be treated by encircling his navel with a leather belt and having two or three people urinate into the belt circle to keep the navel warm. Alternative treatments are to use hot earth in place of urine and encircle the earth with a leather belt, or to break open the bottom of an earthen bowl or che gang (an earthen vessel), press it on the patient's navel, and have many people urinate into the che gang. Take care to prevent leakage of the urine. These are convenient ways of healing if there is no warm water available. If warm water is at hand, it can be used. Since earth and che gang cool off easily, they are not preferred. However, in the summer when sunstroke often occurs, earth and chegang which have been heated by the sun may be used.

第十六节　救溺死方：取灶中灰两石余，以埋人，从头至足。水出七孔，即活。右疗自缢、溺、耙之法，并出自张仲景为之，其意殊绝，殆非常情所及，本草所能关，实救人之大术矣。伤寒家数有耙病，非此遇热之耙。

16. To revive a drowning victim, first bury him from the feet up to the head in a pit filled with

at least two hundred catties of ash from a furnace. If water flows from the seven cavities, the patient will survive.

That the above two remedies for drowning and hanging were both devised by Zhang zhong jing is quite uniquely significant and beyond ordinary understanding. They could not be included in herbals and are truly great life-saving arts. In shanghan patients we frequently encounter heatstroke which is different from the above condition.

第十七节　治马坠及一切筋骨损方。

大黄一两(切浸汤成下),绯帛(如手大烧灰)、乱发(如鸡子大烧灰用)、久用炊单布一尺烧灰,败蒲一握三寸,桃仁四十九个,去皮尖熬,甘草如中指节(炙)。

剉上七味,以童子小便量多少煎汤成,内酒一大盏,次下大黄,去滓,分温三服。先剉败蒲席半领,煎汤浴,衣被盖复,斯须通利数行,痛楚立差,利及浴水赤,勿怪,即瘀血也。

17. The following formulas help a person who has fallen off his horse and treat injured sinews and bones.

1 liang sliced rhubarb soaked in water to produce juice

1 ball human hair the size of an egg burnt to ash

1 hand-size piece red linen burnt to ash

1 foot long used cooking cloth burnt to ash

1 handful (3 inches) worn out acorus mat

1 piece baked licorice, the size of a middle finger, shredded

49 persica seeds with outer skin and apexes removed

Place and decoct all the herbs except rhubarb in a young child's urine; add one big bowl of wine and rhubarb. After discarding the dregs, the decoction is taken warmed in three divided doses. Next, chop and boil half of a worn out mat of acorus and bathe the patient in the water. After washing him, dress him and wrap him with quilts until he urinates several times. The pains will abate immediately. Do not be surprised by the red color of the urine or the bath water; the red comes from extravasated blood.

禽兽鱼虫禁忌并治第二十四

XXIV.

On Treatment of Poisoning from Eating Fowl, Cattle, Hogs, Insects, and Fish

第一节　凡饮食滋味,以养于生,食之有妨,反能为害。自非服药炼液,焉能不饮食乎? 切见时人,不闲调摄,疾疢竞起,若不因食而生,苟全其生,须知切忌者矣,所食之味,有与病相宜,有与身相害,若得宜则益体,害则成疾,以此致危,例皆难疗。凡煮药饮汁以解毒者,虽云救急,不可热饮,诸毒病得热更甚,宜冷饮之。

1. Foods, beverages, and seasonings usually sustain us but sometimes they hurt us. Unlike herbal decoctions, food must be eaten every day, and people who do not partake of healthy diets become susceptible to various kinds of disease. Even though food does not cause disease as such, certain contraindications and compatibilities of foods exist. These should be known in order to maintain proper nutrition. For instance, some foods are beneficial in curing certain diseases while others exacerbate the problem. Beneficial foods promote health; harmful foods injure and weaken the body, making it more prone to disease. An example is an antidote prepared by cooking in a liquid. It should not be drunk hot – even if it is an emergency because heat aggravates toxic action. Usually antidotes should be taken cool. The general rules for eating are many.

第二节　肝病禁辛,心病禁咸,脾病禁酸,肺病禁苦,肾病禁甘。春不食肝,夏不食心,秋不食肺,冬不食肾,四季不食脾。辩曰:春不食肝者,为肝气王,脾气败,若食肝,则又补肝,脾气败尤甚,不可救。又肝王之时,不可以死气入肝,恐伤魂也。若非王时即虚,以肝补之佳,余脏准此。

2. Do not eat acrid foods when afflicted with liver diseases; salty foods, with heart diseases; sour foods, with spleen diseases; bitter foods, with lung diseases; and sweet foods, with kidney diseases, in spring liver should not be eaten; in summer heart should not be eaten; in autumn lung should not be eaten; in winter kidney should not be eaten; in all seasons spleen should not be eat-

en. The reasons for these prohibitions are several. In spring the liver reaches its climax of exuberance and depletes the spleen. The eating of liver augments the exuberance and further depletes the spleen, ultimately leading to an incurable condition. Also, during the liver's exuberant period, the genuine hepatic Qi should not be introduced into the liver, otherwise the soul will be injured. In all except the exuberant season, it is good to supplement the liver with liver. This rule applies to other visceral organs as well.

第三节　凡肝脏,自不可轻啖,自死者弥甚。

3. Do not eat liver from an animal who has died on its own.

第四节　凡心皆为神识所舍,勿食之,使人来生复其报对矣。

4. Because the heart houses spiritual sentience, do not eat it lest the spirit therein take revenge in the ensuing generation.

第五节　凡肉及肝,落地不着尘土者,不可食之。

5. Do not eat flesh and liver that absorb no ash when dropped on the ground.

第六节　猪肉落水浮者,不可食。

6. Do not eat pork that floats on water.

第七节　诸肉及鱼,若狗不食,鸟不啄者,不可食。

7. Do not eat meat and fish which dogs and birds refuse to eat.

第八节　诸肉不干,火炙不动,见水自动者,不可食之。

8. Do not eat moist meat that remains motionless when baked but moves on contact with water.

第九节　肉中有如朱点者,不可食之。

9. Do not eat meat with red spots on it.

第十节　六畜肉热血不断者,不可食之。

10. Do not eat meat of cattle from which hot blood has flowed continuously.

第十一节　父母及身本命肉,食之,令人神魂不安。

11. If a person eats his parents' or his own flesh, he will become spiritually unstable.

第十二节　食肥肉及热羹,不得饮冷水。

12. Do not drink cold water after eating fat meat and a hot broth.

第十三节·诸五脏及鱼,投地尘土不污者,不可食之。

13. Do not eat visceral organs and fish that do not absorb ash when dropped on the ground.

第十四节　秽饭、馁肉、臭鱼,食之皆伤人。

14. Spoiled rice, meat from a starved animal, and stinking fish will injure those who eat them.

第十五节　自死肉,口闭者,不可食之。

15. Do not eat meat from animals that have died with their mouths closed.

第十六节　六畜自死,皆疫死,则有毒,不可食之。

16. Poultry and cattle that die by themselves all die of plague; their meat is poisonous and should not be eaten.

第十七节　兽自死,北首及伏地者,食之杀人。

17. Animals that die in a prostrate position with their head facing north should not be eaten; the meat will kill the eater.

第十八节　食生肉,饱饮乳,变成白虫;一作血蛊。

18. Eating raw meat and drinking milk to the full produces white worms or Xuegu (blood

worms).

第十九节　疫死牛肉,食之令病洞下,亦致坚积,宜利药下之。

19. Eating beef from plague-stricken oxen will cause severe diarrhea and hardening tumors; the afflicted should be purged.

第二十节　脯藏米瓮中,有毒,及经夏食之,发肾病。

20. Dried meat preserved in an earthen jar containing rice is poisonous. It will injure the kidneys if eaten after having been stored for one summer.

第二十一节　治(食)自死六畜肉中毒方：黄蘗屑,捣服方寸匕。

21. An antidote for poisoning from eating poultry and cattle that have died by themselves is: Pound chips of phellodendron into powder and take at a dose of about one fangcunbi.

第二十二节　治食郁肉漏脯中毒方：郁肉,密器盖之,隔宿者是也。漏脯,茅屋漏下,沾着者是也。烧犬屎,酒服方寸匕,每服人乳汁亦良。饮生韭汁三升,亦得。

22. A treatment for poisoning resulting from eating meat kept overnight in a hermetic container, or dried meat that has been stored under a grass cottage and contaminated by the water leaking through the grass roof, is: Burn dog feces and take one fangcunbi of it along with wine or human milk. An alternativeis to drink 3 sheng of fresh leek juice.

第二十三节　治黍米中藏干脯,食之中毒方：大豆浓煮汁,饮数升即解。亦治诸肉漏脯等毒。

23. A treatment for poisoning from meat stored in millet is: Cook soya beans until a thick juice is produced; several sheng of the juice will detoxify the poison. This formula also treats poisoning from fox meat or from dried meat that has been contaminated by leaking water.

第二十四节　治食生肉中毒方：掘地深三尺,取其下土三升,以水五升煮数沸,澄清汁,饮一升,即愈。

24. A formula for treating poisoning from eating raw meat is: Dig 3 feet into the ground to obtain 3 sheng of earth from the lower layer. Place the earth in 5 sheng of water and decoct. After the

decoction has settled and cleared, drink 1 sheng of the clear, supernatant solution.

第二十五节 治(食)六畜鸟兽肝中毒方：水浸豆豉,绞取汁,服数升愈。

25．A treatment for poisoning from eating the liver of poultry and cattle is: Pickle soya bean relish with water, then strain. Take several sheng of the juice at a time.

第二十六节 马脚无夜眼者,不可食之。

26．Do not eat meat from a horse that does not have calosities on the knees.

第二十七节 食酸马肉,不饮酒,则杀人。

27．Eating sour horse meat without drinking wine will belethal.

第二十八节 马肉不可热食,伤人心。

28．The eating of hot horse meat will injure the heart.

第二十九节 马鞍下肉,食之杀人。

29．Horse flesh from beneath the saddle is lethal when eaten.

第三十节 白马黑头者,不可食之。

30．Do not eat the meat of a horse with a white bodyand a black head.

第三十一节 白马青蹄者,不可食之。

31．Do not eat the meat of a horse with a white bodyand blue hoofs.

第三十二节 马肉狍肉共食,饱醉卧,大忌。

32．It is taboo to eat one's fill of horse and hog meat together with wine to the point of drunkenness and sleep.

第三十三节 驴马肉合猪肉食之,成霍乱。

33．The eating of a mixture of horse, mule, and hog meat causes cholera.

第三十四节　马肝及毛,不可妄食,中毒害人。

34．Profligate eating of horse liver and hair causes poisoning.

第三十五节　治马肝毒中人未死方:雄鼠屎二七粒,末之,水和服,日再服。屎尖者是。又方:人垢,取方寸匕,服之佳。

35．A treatment for poisoning by horse liver is: Grind 27 male mouse droppings (the pointed ones) into powder and take with water twice daily; one fangcunbi of human dandruff may be substituted.

第三十六节　治食马肉中毒欲死方:香豉二两,杏仁三两。
上二味,蒸一食顷熟,杵之服,日再服。又方:煮芦根汁,饮之良。

36．A treatment for poisoning from eating horse meat is: Steam 2 liang of soya bean relish and 3 liang of apricot seeds together until well cooked; then pound and take twice daily. Or else drink the juice from boiled roots of phragmites.

第三十七节　疫死牛,或目赤,或黄,食之大忌。

37．It is taboo to eat the meat of plague-stricken oxen or oxen with red or yellow eyes.

第三十八节　牛肉共猪肉食之,必作寸白虫。

38．Eating a mixture of beef and pork causes cun pai chong (inch-long white worms).

第三十九节　青牛肠,不可合犬肉食之。

39．Do not eat the intestines of a black ox with dog meat.

第四十节　牛肺从三月至五月,其中有虫如马尾,割去勿食,食则损人。

40．From March to May ox lungs develop worms that look like horse tails. Do not eat lungs so infested; cut them away; they will cause much harm.

第四十一节　牛、羊、猪肉,皆不得以椿木、桑木蒸炙,食之令人腹内生虫。

41. Do not eat beef, mutton, or pork that has been cooked or broiled over a fire made from the wood of paper mulberry(Broussonetia kasinoki) or the wood of white mulberry (Moms alba); meats so prepared will produce abdominal worms.

第四十二节　啖蛇牛肉杀人,何以知之? 啖蛇者,毛发向后顺者,是也。

42. The meat of an ox that has eaten snakes will kill the man who eats it. How can we identify such an ox? The hair on an ox that eats snakes grows backward.

第四十三节　治啖蛇牛肉食之欲死方:饮人乳汁一升,立愈。又方:以泔洗头,饮一升,愈。牛肚细切,以水一斗,煮取一升,暖饮之,大汗出者愈。

43. The treatments for poisoning from eating the meat of an ox that has eaten snakes are: ① Drink one sheng of human milk. ② Wash the head with the water that has been used to wash rice and drink one sheng of the water that has been used to wash the head. ③ Cut an ox's stomach into fine pieces and cook in 10 sheng of water until one sheng remains; drink the liquid warmed. The afflicted will recover after profusely perspiring.

第四十四节　治食牛肉中毒方:甘草煮汁饮之,即解。

44. For poisoning from the eating of beef decoct licorice and drink the juice.

第四十五节　羊肉其有宿热者,不可食之。

45. Do not eat mutton that remains hot overnight.

第四十六节　羊肉不可共生鱼、酪食之,害人。

46. Mutton eaten with raw fish broth will harm the eater.

第四十七节　羊蹄甲中有珠子白者,名羊悬筋,食之令人癫。

47. White spots like beads in the hoofs of a goat are known as yang xuan jin (goat's hanging sinew); meat from such a goat causes epilepsy if eaten.

第四十八节　白羊黑头,食其脑,作肠痈。

48. The eating of the brain of a white goat with a black head will cause intestinal carbuncles.

第四十九节　羊肝共生椒食之,破人五脏。

49. The eating of goat liver with raw pepper destroys the viscera.

第五十节　猪肉共羊肝和食之,令人心闷。

50. The eating of pork with goat liver causes a depressive feeling in the heart.

第五十一节　猪肉以生胡荽同食,烂人脐。

51. The eating of pork with raw coriander erodes the navel.

第五十二节　猪脂不可合梅子食之。

52. Lard should not be eaten with prunes.

第五十三节　猪肉和葵食之,少气。

53. The eating of pork with sunflowers depletes vitality.

第五十四节　鹿人(肉)不可和蒲白作羹,食之发恶疮。

54. The eating of a broth made of deer meat and the white bark of acorus produces noxious sores.

第五十五节　麋脂及梅李子,若妊妇食之,令子青盲,男子伤精。

55. The eating of the fat of Akes machilis with prunes by a pregnant woman causes glaucoma in her child. When eaten by a man, it causes injury to his sperm.

第五十六节　獐肉不可合虾及生菜、梅、李果食之;皆病人。

56. Do not eat the meat of roe deer (Moschus chinico) with shrimp, raw vegetables, prunes, plums, or fruits. It will make the eater sick.

第五十七节 痼疾人不可食熊肉,令终身不愈。

57. One who has a chronic disease should not eat bear meat or he will have the disease all his life.

第五十八节 白犬自死,不出舌者,食之害人。

58. The eating of the meat of a white dog which has died on its own without sticking out its tongue will harm the eater.

第五十九节 食狗鼠余,令人发瘘疮。

59. The eating of food which a dog and mouse have partially eaten produces fistulas.

第六十节 治食犬肉不消成病方:治食犬肉不消,心下坚,或腹胀,口干大渴,心急发热,妄语如狂,或洞下方杏仁一升,(合皮熟研用)以沸汤三升和,取汁,分三服,利下肉片,大验。

60. The formula for treating indigestion from eating dog meat, the accompanying symptoms of which are hardness beneath the heart, abdominal distention, dry mouth, severe thirst, an urgent feeling in the heart with fever, manic delirium, and diarrhea – is this: Cook one sheng of apricot seeds, with the skin on, and then grind them into powder. Combine the powder with 3 sheng of boiling water, stir well, strain, and take the solution warmed in three portions. If the patient discharges the ingested meat through diarrhea, the formula has been effective.

第六十一节 妇人妊娠,不可食兔肉、山羊肉,及鳖、鸡、鸭,令子无声音。

61. A pregnant woman should not eat the meat of the rabbit, goat, turtle, chicken, or duck as these produce muteness in the expected child.

第六十二节 兔肉不可合白鸡肉食之,令人面发黄。

62. The eating of rabbit meat with white chicken meat causes yellowing of the face.

第六十三节　兔肉着干姜食之，成霍乱。

63．The eating of rabbit meat with dried ginger causes cholera．

第六十四节　凡鸟自死，口不闭，翅不合者，不可食之。

64．Do not eat a bird that has died by itself with its mouth open and its wmgs spread．

第六十五节　诸禽肉，肝青者，食之杀人。

65．The eating of a bird with a green liver will kill the eater．

第六十六节　鸡有六翮四距者，不可食之。

66．Do not eat chicken with six web less spaces between the claws and four spurs．

第六十七节　乌鸡白首者，不可食之。

67．Do not eat a black chicken with a white head．

第六十八节　鸡不可共葫蒜食之，滞气。

68．Chicken or eggs eaten with garlic impedes vitality．

第六十九节　山鸡不可合鸟兽肉食之。

69．Do not eat pheasant with other bird or animal meat．

第七十节　雉肉久食之，令人瘦。

70．The eating of pheasant for a long time causes emaciation．

第七十一节　鸭卵不可合鳖肉食之。

71．Do not eat duck eggs with fresh water turtle meat．

第七十二节　妇人妊娠食雀肉，令子淫乱无耻。

72. A pregnant woman who eats sparrow meat will give birth to a lustful child.

第七十三节　雀肉不可合李子食之。

73. Do not eat sparrow meat with plums.

第七十四节　燕肉勿食,入水为蛟龙所啖。

74. Do not eat swallow meat. The eater of swallow meat will be eaten by a scaly dragon (crocodile) when he enters the water where the dragon lives.

第七十五节　鸟兽有中毒箭死者,其肉有毒,解之方大豆煮汁及盐汁服之解。

75. Birds and animals that die of arrow poisoning have poison in their meat. For an antidote, cook soya beans until reduced to juice and take the juice with saline water.

第七十六节　鱼头正白,如连珠至脊上,食之杀人。

76. The eating of a fish with pure white spots extending from the head to the spine like a string of beads will kill the eater.

第七十七节　鱼头无腮者,不可食之,杀人。

77. The eating of a fish without gills in the head will kill the eater.

第七十八节　鱼无肠胆者,不可食之,三年阴不起,女子绝生。

78. The eating of a fish without intestines and gall will cause impotence in males for three years and infecundity in females.

第七十九节　鱼头似有角者,不可食之。

79. Do not eat a fish with a horn-like growth on its head.

第八十节　鱼目合者,不可食之。

80. Do not eat a fish which has closed eyes.

第八十一节 六甲日,勿食鳞甲之物。

81. On the six jia days (days whose names bear the first celestial stem, jia) do not eat meat from animals that have scales or shells.

第八十二节 鱼不可合鸡肉食之。

82. Do not eat fish with chicken.

第八十三节 鱼不得合鸬鹚肉食之。

83. Do not eat fish with egret.

第八十四节 鲤鱼鲊,不可合小豆藿食之,其子不可合猪肝食之,害人。

84. Do not eat preserved carp with the tender leaves of small beans; carp eggs should not be eaten with hog liver, otherwise the eater will be harmed.

第八十五节 鲤鱼不可合犬肉食之。

85. Do not eat carp with dog meat.

第八十六节 鲤鱼不可合猴雉肉食之。一云不可合猪肝食。

86. Do not eat bastard carp with monkey and pheasant meat. (Another saying holds not to eat bastard carp with hog liver)

第八十七节 鲲鱼合鹿肉生食,令人筋甲缩。

87. The eating of raw sheat fish. with raw deer meat may produce muscle atrophy.

第八十八节 青鱼鲊,不可合生葫荽及生葵并麦中食之。

88. Do not eat preserved mackerel with raw coriander, malva, and wheat.

第八十九节　鳅、鳝不可合白犬血食之。

89. Do not eat the meat of Misgurus anguilicandatus and yellow eel with a white dog's blood.

第九十节　龟肉不可合酒、果子食之。

90. Do not eat turtle with wine and pickled fruits.

第九十一节　鳖目凹陷者,及厌下有王字形者,不可食之。

91. Do not eat a fresh water turtle that has sunken eyes and a figure "王" beneath its cheeks.

第九十二节　其肉不得合鸡、鸭子食之。

92. Do not eat the meat of fresh water turtle with chicken or duck eggs.

第九十三节　龟、鳖肉不可合苋菜食之。

93. Do not eat turtle with Amaranthus mangostanus.

第九十四节　虾无须,及腹下通黑,煮之反白者,不可食之。

94. Do not eat shrimp without tentacles or with a black color covering the entire abdomen which turns white after cooking.

第九十五节　食脍,饮乳酪,令人腹中生虫为瘕。

95. Thinly sliced meat eaten with cheese will cause the growth of worms and development of tumors in the abdomen.

第九十六节　鲙食之,在心胸间不化,吐复不出,速下除之,久成癥病,治之方：橘皮一两,大黄二两,朴硝二两。
上三味,以水一大升,煮至小升,顿服即消。

96. Thinly sliced fish that becomes lodged between the heart and diaphragm and can not be vomited should be purged at once, otherwise an abdominal tumor will develop. The formula called for contains 1 liang of citrus, 2 liang of rhubarb, and 2 liang of mirabilitum. Boil the ingredients in

1 big sheng of water until 1 small sheng remains. Take all in one draft. The obstruction will be resolved at once.

第九十七节　食鲙多不消,结为癥病。治之方：马鞭草。
上一味,捣汁饮之,或以姜叶汁饮之一升,亦消。又可服吐药吐之。

97. Thinly sliced fish is often indigestible and produces abdominal tumors. They can be treated with the following formula: Verbena pounded into juice, or else 1 sheng of the juice from ginger leaves. Both formulas dissolve tumors. An emetic may also be prescribed.

第九十八节　食鱼后食毒,两种烦乱,治之方：橘皮。
浓煎汁服之,即解。

98. A formula for treating vexation and upset after eating fish or toxic foods is orange peel decocted into a thick juice. It will alleviate the poisoning at once.

第九十九节　食鳀鲙鱼中毒方：芦根煮汁服之,即解。

99. For treating poisoning from eating puffers drink the decocted juice of phragmites (common reed) root. It will dissolve the poison at once.

第一〇〇节　蟹目相向,足斑目赤者,不可食之。

100. Do not eat a crab with crossed and red eyes and maculated legs.

第一〇一节　食蟹中毒治之方：紫苏。
煮汁饮之三升。紫苏子捣汁饮之,亦良。
又方：冬瓜汁饮二升,食冬瓜亦可。

101. For treating poisoning from eating crabs, cook perfita and drink the decoction; or pound perilla seeds into juice and drink; or drink 2 sheng of gourd melon juice; or eat gourd melon.

第一〇二节　凡蟹未遇霜,多毒,其熟者乃可食之。

102. Crabs that have not lived past the frost season are poisonous; cooking makes them edible.

第一〇三节　一蜘蛛落食中,有毒,勿食之。

103. Do not eat foods on which a spider has fallen.

第一〇四节　凡蜂、蝇、虫、蚁等多集食上，食之致瘘。

104. Do not eat foods on which bees, flies, and ants are clustered. Eating such foods causes fistula.

果实菜谷禁忌并治第二十五

XXV.

On Pulse Syndrome Complex and Treatment of Poisoning from Eating Fruits, Vegetables, and Cereals

第一节　果子生食生疮。

1. The eating of raw fruit can produce sores.

第二节　果子落地经宿,虫蚁食之者,人大忌食之。

2. Fruit that has fallen to the ground and lain there for one night and that has been eaten by insects or ants is forbidden to humans.

第三节　生米停留多日,有损处,食之伤人。

3. Raw rice that has been stored for a number of days and shows sign of decay in some portion will injure the eater.

第四节　桃子多食令人热,仍不得入水浴,令人病淋沥寒热病。

4. The excessive eating of peaches causes heat. The eater should not then bathe himself in water lest he develop uninary stuttering, chills, and fever.

第五节　杏酪不熟伤人。

5. An insufficiently cooked gruel made of apricots injures the eater.

第六节　梅多食,坏人齿。

6. The excessive eating of prunes injures the teeth.

第七节　李不可多食,令人胪胀。

7. The excessive eating of plums causes abdominal distention.

第八节　林擒不可多食,令人百脉弱。

8. The excessive eating of apples weakens the pulse.

第九节　橘柚多食,令人口爽,不知五味。

9. The excessive eating of oranges or grapefruits numbs the mouth and causes loss of taste.

第十节　梨不可多食,令人寒中,金疮、产妇亦不宜食。

10. Pears should not be eaten excessively, otherwise the eater will develop a chill stomach. Patients with wounds from metals or postpartum women are also advised to avoid pears.

第十一节　樱桃、杏多食,伤筋骨。

11. The excessive eating of cherries or apricots injures the sinews and bones.

第十二节　安石榴不可多食,损人肺。

12. Pomegranates should not be eaten excessively because they will injure the lungs.

第十三节　胡桃不可多食,令人动痰饮。

13. Walnuts eaten excessively induce water and sputum problems.

第十四节　生枣多食,令人热渴气胀。寒热羸瘦者,弥不可食,伤人。

14. Raw jujube eaten excessively causes fever, thirst, and Qi distention; it especially injures chilled, feverish, weak, and emaciated people.

第十五节　食诸果中毒治之方：猪骨烧灰。

上一味,末之,水服方寸匕。亦治马肝、漏脯等毒。

15. For treating poisoning from eating fruits: grind burnt pig bones into a powder and take one fangcunbi at a time. The formula also treats poisoning from eating horse liver or dried meat contaminated by water leaking from a roof.

第十六节　木耳赤色,及仰生者,勿食。

16. Do not eat auricularia (Jew's ear) that is red and grows in a supine position.

第十七节　菌仰卷及赤色者,不可食。

17. Do not eat red fungi that grow curled up in a supine position.

第十八节　食诸菌中毒,闷乱欲死,治之方：人粪汁,饮一升。土浆,饮一二升。大豆浓煮汁饮之。服诸吐利药,并解。

18. For treating poisoning from eating fungi that has caused a depressive and violent sensation so severe that the victim feels as if he were going to die, drink a mixture of one sheng of human feces juice, 1 to 2 sheng of soil water, and thick soya juice (prepared by boiling soya beans). Emetics or purgatives also may help.

第十九节　食枫柱菌而哭不止,治之以前方。

19. The preceeding formula also helps incessant laughing from the eating of fungi growing on a maple tree.

第二十节　误食野芋,烦毒欲死,治之以前方。

20. The preceding formula also treats life-threatening poisoning from eating wild taro.

第二十一节　蜀椒闭口者有毒,误食之,戟人咽喉,气病欲绝,或吐下白沫,身体痹冷,急治之方肉桂煎汁饮之,多饮冷水一二升,或食蒜,或饮地浆,或浓煮豉汁饮之,并解。

21. Zanthoxylum fruits with closed carpels are poisonous; mistaken ingestion irritates the throat and causes life-threatening Qi disease. The eater will vomit white froth and become numb and

chilled. Give the following at once: Decocted cinnamon juice with 1 to 2 shengs of cool water; or garlic; or soil water; or the thick juice of soya bean relish.

第二十二节　正月勿食生葱,令人面生游风。二月勿食蓼,伤人肾。三月勿食小蒜,伤人志性。四月、八月勿食胡荽,伤人神。五月勿食韭,令人乏气力。五月五日勿食一切生菜,发百病。六月、七月勿食茱萸,伤神气。八月、九月勿食姜,伤人神。十月勿食椒,损人心,伤心脉。十一月、十二月勿食薤,令人多涕唾。

22. In the first month of each year of the Chinese lunar calendar, do not eat raw scallion; it will cause eczema on the face.

In the second month, do not eat red smartweed (Polygonum hydropiper); it will injure the kidneys.

In the third month, do not eat "lesser garlic"; it will injure the will and temper.

In the fourth and eighth months, do not eat coriander; it will injure the spirit.

In the fifth month, do not eat leek; it will exhaust the vitality.

On the fifth day of the fifth month, do not eat any raw vegetables; they will cause disease.

In the sixth and seventh months, do not eat evodia; it will injure the spirit and Qi.

In the eighth and ninth months, do not eat ginger; it will injure one's spirit.

In the tenth month, do not eat pepper; it will injure the heart and cardiovascular system.

In the eleventh and twelfth months, do not eat Chinese chive (Allium bakeri); it will cause profuse snivel and saliva.

第二十三节　四季勿食生葵,令人饮食不化,发百病。非但食中,药中皆不可用,深宜慎之。

23. In all seasons, raw malva will cause indigestion and all sorts of diseases. It should not be eaten with other foods or used as an ingredient in a medical formula. One must be aware of this.

第二十四节　时病差未健,食生菜,手足必肿。

24. The eating of raw vegetables when still recovering from an epidemic will cause the extremities to swell.

第二十五节　夜食生菜,不利人。

25. Eating raw vegetables at night is detrimental.

第二十六节　十月勿食被霜生菜,令人面无光,目涩,心痛,腰疼,或发心疟。疟发时,手足十指爪皆青,困委。

26. In the tenth month, do not eat vegetables that have been subject to frost or else one will lose facial gloss, suffer from eye irritation, and develop pain in the heart, lumbago, or cardiac malaria which on seizure manifests blueness and weakness in the fingers and toes.

第二十七节　葱、韭初生芽者,食之伤人心气。

27. Eating the new sprouts of scallion and leek injures the heart Qi.

第二十八节　饮白酒,食生韭,令人病增。

28. Drinking white wine and eating raw leek aggravates existent diseases.

第二十九节　生葱不可共蜜食之,杀人。独颗蒜弥忌。

29. Do not eat raw scallion, especially mono corm scallion, with honey; it will kill the eater.

第三十节　枣和生葱食之,令人病。

30. The eating of jujube with raw scallion makes the eater sick.

第三十一节　生葱和雄鸡、雉、白犬肉食之,令人七窍经年流血。

31. The eating of raw scallion with cock, pheasant, or white dog causes the seven cavities to bleed incessantly all yearlong.

第三十二节　食糖、蜜后四日内食生葱、韭,令人心痛。

32. The eating of raw scallion or leek four days after previous ingestion of honcy causes heart pain.

第三十三节　夜食诸姜、蒜、葱等,伤人心。

33. The eating of ginger, garlic, or scallion at night injures the heart.

第三十四节　芜菁根多食,令人气胀。

34. The eating of too much of the root of rapeseed (Brassica rapadepressa) causes distention of Qi.

第三十五节　薤不可共牛肉作羹,食之成瘕病,韭亦然。

35. Allium bakeri cooked with beef to produce a broth causes tumors. This is also true of leek.

第三十六节　蓴多食,动痔疾。

36. The eating of too much of brasenia schreberi induces hemorrhoids.

第三十七节　野苣不可同蜜食之,作内痔。

37. Wild alfalfa eaten with honey causes internal hemorrhoids.

第三十八节　白苣不可共酪同食,作䘌虫。

38. White alfalfa eaten with cheese produces ni worms (small worms).

第三十九节　黄瓜食之,发热病。

39. The eating of curcumis sativus produces fever.

第四十节　葵心不可食,伤人,叶尤冷,黄背赤茎者,勿食之。

40. The heart portion of malva (Chinese mallow) injures the eater. The leaves of malva are especially cold. Do not eat the species with yellow on the back of leaves and red stems.

第四十一节　胡荽久食之,令人多忘。

41. Coriander eaten for a prolonged time causes amnesia.

第四十二节　病人不可食胡荽及黄花菜(菜)。

42. A sick individual should not eat coriander and wild lettuce (Lactuca thumbe giana Max).

第四十三节　芋不可多食,动病。

43. Taro eaten excessively induces disease.

第四十四节　妊妇食姜,令子余指。

44. A pregnant woman who eats ginger will give birth to a child with extra fingers.

第四十五节　蓼多食,发心痛。

45. The excessive eating of polygonum hyclropiper produces heart pain.

第四十六节　蓼和生鱼食之,令人夺气,阴咳疼痛。

46. The eating of polygonum hydropiper with raw fish exhausts Qi and causes pudendal (clitoris) aching.

第四十七节　芥菜不可共兔肉食之,成恶邪病。

47. The eating of brassica juncea with rabbit meat causes noxious disease.

第四十八节　小蒜多食,伤人心力。

48. Excessive eating of "lesser garlic" injures the mental power.

第四十九节　食躁或躁方:豉浓煮汁饮之。

49. For treating irritation with occasional nausea after eating, cook soya bean relish until it is a thick juice; then drink the juice.

第五十节　误食钩吻杀人解之方:钩吻与芹菜相似,误食之杀人,解之方。
荠苨八两。
上一味,水六升,煮取二升,分温二服。

50. The mistaken ingestion of Gouwen, which resembles celery, kills the eater. The antidote

is the same as for the ingestion of evodia with celery or place 8 liang of harebell in 6 sheng of water and decoct until 2 sheng remains. Drink warmed in two divided portions.

第五十一节　治误食水茛菪中毒方：菜中有水茛菪,叶圆而光,有毒。误食之,令人狂乱,状如中风,或吐血,治之方甘草煮汁服之,即解。

51. Among vegetables, the one known as shui langtang with round glossy leaves is poisonous. When eaten by mistake, it causes erratic behavior or even violence, as though apoplectic, or hematemesis. The antidote is decocted licorice juice. This relieves the symptoms at once.

第五十二节　治食芹菜中龙精毒方：(原缺)春秋二时,龙带精入芹菜中,人偶食之为病。发时手青腹满,痛不可忍,名蛟龙病,治之方硬糖二三斤。
上一味,日两度服之,吐出如晰蜴三五枚,差。

52. In the spring and autumn the dragon delivers his spermon to the oenanthe. When eaten by accident, the plant produces a disease that manifests blue hands, abdominal swelling, and unbearable pain. The condition, known as "scaly dragon (crocodile) disease," requires the antidote of 2 to 3 sheng of solid sugar (or sweet jelly made from glutinous rice) taken twice daily. Once the patient vomits three to five lizard-like reptiles, he is well.

第五十三节　食苦瓠中毒治之方：黎穰煮汁,数服之,解。

53. The treatment for poisoning from the ingestion of calabash is to cook millet stems until a juice; then drink the juice. Several solutions may be required.

第五十四节　扁豆,寒热者不可食之。

54. Those who have chills or fever should not eat hyacinth bean.

第五十五节　久食小豆,令人枯燥。

55. The eating of red mung beans for a long time causes aridity and emaciation.

第五十六节　食大豆屑,忌啖猪肉。

56. Do not eat pork after eating soya bean chips.

第五十七节　大麦久食。令人作癣。

57. Prolonged eating of barley causes one to develop scabies.

第五十八节　白黍米不可同饴、蜜食,亦不可合葵食之。

58. Do not eat white millet with maltose, honey, or malva.

第五十九节　荍(荞)麦面多食之,令人发落。

59. The frequent eating of the flour of buckwheat (Fagopyrum esculentum) causes the hair to fall out.

第六十节　盐多食,伤人肺。

60. Eating large amounts of table salt injures the lungs.

第六十一节　食冷物,冰人齿。

61. The eating of cold foods chills the teeth.

第六十二节　食热物,勿饮冷水。

62. Do not drink cold water after eating hot food.

第六十三节　饮酒,食生苍耳,令人心痛。

63. Drinking liquor and eating raw cocklebur causes heart pain.

第六十四节　夏月大醉汗流,不得冷水洗着身,及使扇,即成病。

64. In the summer a severely drunk person who is sweating should not wash himself with cold water or use a fan to cool himself, otherwise he will get sick.

第六十五节　饮酒,大忌炙腹背,令人肠结。

65. Moxibustion performed on the back or abdomen of a person who has drunk liquor causes

intestinal obstruction.

第六十六节　醉后勿饱食,发寒热。

66. After becoming drunk, a person should not eat to fullness, otherwise he will have chills and fever.

第六十七节　饮酒食猪肉,卧秫稻穰中则发黄。

67. Lying on the stems of glutinous rice after drinking liquor and eating pork causes yellowing.

第六十八节　食饴,多饮酒,大忌。

68. Do not drink liquor after eating large quantities of maltose.

第六十九节　凡水及酒,照见人影动者,不可饮之。

69. Do not drink water and wine that reflect moving images.

第七十节　醋和酪食之,令人血瘕。

70. The eating of vinegar and cheese together produces hematoma.

第七十一节　食白米粥,勿食生苍耳,成走疰。

71. The eating of raw cocklebur after eating white rice congee causes wind paralysis (moving pain, rheumatism).

第七十二节　食甜粥已,食盐即吐。

72. The eating of table salt after eating sweet rice congee causes vomiting.

第七十三节　犀角筋搅饮食,沫出及浇地坟起者,食之杀人。

73. Foods or beverages that produce froth when stirred with a rhinoceros horn and form a heap when poured onto the ground will kill if eaten.

第七十四节　饮食中毒,烦满,治之方：苦参三两,苦酒一升半。
上二味,煮三沸,三上三下,服之,吐食出,即差。或以水煮亦得。又方犀角汤亦佳。

74. The treatment for the distress and distention caused by food poisoning is this: Bring 3 liang of sophora and 1.5 sheng of vinegar to a boil three times; then drink. Once the ingested food is vomited, the patient heals. The ingredients may be boiled in water.

Another formula is Xi-jiao-tang (Rhinoceros Combination) prepared by grinding rhinoceros horn in water.

第七十五节　贪食、食多不消,心腹坚满痛,治之方：盐一升,水三升。
上二味,煮令盐消,分三服,当吐出食,便差。

75. For treating hardening, swelling, and pain in the heart and abdomen as a consequence of indigestion due to gluttony, boil 2 sheng of table salt in 3 sheng of water until the salt completely dissolves. Drink in three divided doses. As soon as the person vomits, he heals.

第七十六节　矾石,生入腹,破人心肝,亦禁水。

76. Raw alum ingested will destroy the heart and liver. The drinking of water afterward is forbidden.

第七十七节　商陆,以水服,杀人。

77. Poke weed or pokeberry taken along with water will kill the one who takes it.

第七十八节　亭苈子傅头疮、药成入脑,杀人。

78. Woodsdraba seeds applied as a paste to head sores will penetrate the brain and kill the patient.

第七十九节　水银入人耳,及六畜等,皆死。以金银着耳边,水银则吐。

79. If mercury enters the ears of human beings or animals, death will occur. Gold or silver on the ears draws out the mercury.

第八十节　苦练无子者,杀人。

80. Melia that does not bear fruit kills people.

第八十一节　凡诸毒,多是假毒以投,不知时,宜煮甘草荠苨汁饮之,通除诸毒药。

81. Poison injures the vitality. When one thinks he has been poisoned, he should immediately drink a juice prepared from licorice and harebell. It counteracts all kinds of poison.